KETO DIET

The Ultimate Keto Diet Meal Plan For A Rapid Weight Loss

SERIES book 3 of 6

By Robert Smith

are for clarifying purposes only and are owned by the owners themselves s, not affiliated with this document.

Table of Content

Introduction

In this technological era, it is quite important to take good care of one's health because of change in environment due to unrestricted depletion of natural resources and production of harmful waste products has contributed to the existence of a number of novel lethal viruses and diseases. On the flip side, humans are becoming more ignorant regarding maintaining their health due to hectic routines. Without any discrimination on a financial basis, everyone is so busy performing routine tasks that they find it hard to make out some time to focus on their health. Meanwhile, according to doctors, nowadays, the ratio of patients suffering from obesity is quite high compared to other diseases. A patient is afflicted with obesity when he eats too much and follows an irregular eating routine. Also, lack of physical exercise results in obesity because when a person eats any meal containing fat and other nutrients that are supposed to deliver energy to the body gets stored in his body in the form of fats because they are not used for extracting energy. These fats keep accumulating inside the body because a person does not participate in any activity that needs an excess of energy for which these fats are used; this results in obesity and increases in weight. There is a fix to this problem. Recently, scientists have proposed a Keto diet for patients suffering from Obesity and who want to lose weight. The Keto diet involves restricting carbohydrates and keeping protein consumption at a moderate level while increasing the fat intake. The basic principle is that when a person eats fats, it will provide a quick energy source; hence, fats will break down into fuel for the body. This will lead to the conversion of fats into a fuel source, and with the passage of time, more and more stored fats are converted into fuel for the body hence getting rid of extra weight from the body. While discussing the keto diet, it is a complete diet plan in which different meals are proposed whose constituents are quantized according to the above-mentioned principle of keeping the high-fat contents while keeping protein intake moderate and restricting the carbohydrate consumption. In this book, a complete keto diet plan is discussed that is easy to adopt with maximum effectiveness. However, usually, beginners find it demanding to switch from their tasty and delicious meals to new a completely new diet. In the keto diet, individuals are free to keep their favorite dishes with controlled carbs, and such recipes are provided in this book. It is also important to follow the Keto diet plan religiously to attain the desired outcome in the minimum possible time period; otherwise, it can result in an unhealthy experience for your body with some serious side effects. However, patients who adopt this keto diet wholeheartedly find it a completely different lifestyle with sound mental and physical health.

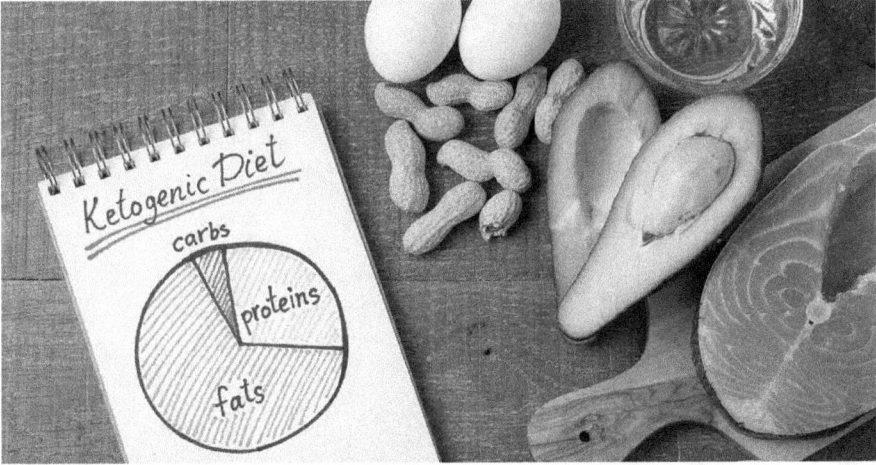

Chapter 1: Breakfast Recipes

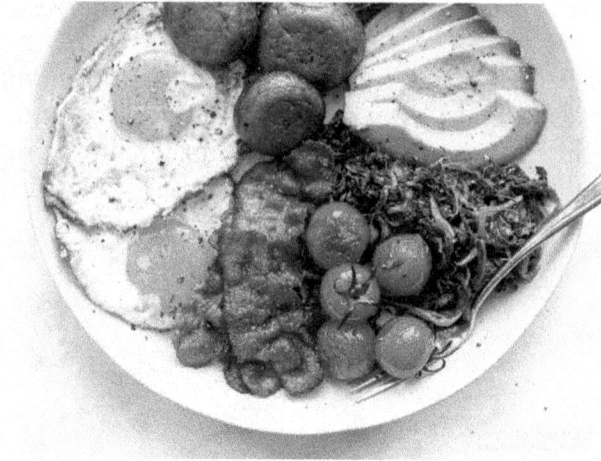

1. Cheesy Bread Bake

Ready in: 20 mins

Servings: 5

Difficulty: Easy

INGREDIENTS

- One loaf of any bread

- 1 cup mozzarella cheese (shredded)

- ¼ cup butter

- 2 cups cheddar cheese (shredded)

- ¼ cup of mayonnaise

- Two cloves minced garlic

- ¼ cup green onion, finely chopped

DIRECTIONS

1. Mix garlic and butter in a bowl.

2. Mix green onion and cheese separately in a bowl, and then add mayonnaise to it.

3. Add this mixture of cheese into butter and garlic mixture.

4. Spread the mixture on the bread loaf.

5. Preheat the broiler and place bread for 4 to 5 mins.

6. Let it cool for 5 mins and then slice it with a knife

7. Serve it.

NUTRITION: Calories: 199 cal Fat: 14 g Protein: 6 g Carbs: 25 g

2. Cocoa Oatmeal

Ready in: 8 minutes

Servings: 1

Difficulty: Easy

INGREDIENTS

- ½ tsp vanilla extract

- ¾ cup oats

- Sea salt to taste

- 1 1/3 cup almond milk

- 2 tsp brown sugar

- ½ sliced banana

- 2tpsp cocoa powder

DIRECTIONS

1. Combine all the ingredients in a mixing bowl.

2. Cook it for 5 to 8 minutes at the medium flame with frequent stirring.

3. Pour it in a bowl and enjoy it.

NUTRITION: Calories: 360 cal Fat: 9 g Protein: 12 g Carbs: 67 g

3. Cheddar Hash Browns

Ready in: 50 minutes

Servings: 11

Difficulty: Medium

INGREDIENTS

- 1 cup parmesan cheese, grated

- 30 oz. hash brown, shredded and frozen potatoes

- 2 cups cheddar cheese, shredded

- Two cans of condensed cream (potato soup)

- 2 cups of sour cream

DIRECTIONS

1. Take half of the cheddar cheese and all the remaining ingredients in a mixing bowl.

2. Pour this mixture into a baking dish.

3. Now add the left amount of cheddar cheese.

4. Heat oven to 340° and bake it for 43 mins.

5. Leave it for 10 mins before serving.

NUTRITION: Calories: 305 cal Fat: 17 g Protein: 11 g Carbs: 22 g

4. Banana and Blueberry Oats

Prep in: 10 minutes

Chill in: 8 hour

Servings: 1

Difficulty: difficult

INGREDIENTS

- 1 tsp vanilla

- ½ cup oats

- 1/3 cup sliced banana

- ½ cup milk

- ½ cup blueberries

DIRECTIONS

1. Mix vanilla, milk, and oats in a bowl.

2. Add blueberries and banana layers over it.

3. Refrigerate it for 8 hours.

4. Serve and enjoy.

NUTRITION: Calories: 320 cal Fat: 5 g Protein: 13 g Carbs: 65 g

5. Trout Frittata

Ready in: 25 minutes

Servings: 5

Difficulty: Easy

INGREDIENTS

- ½ tsp salt

- ¼ cup basil leaves

- Eight eggs

- 4 oz. trout

- ½ cup cream, heavy

- Ten sliced tomatoes

- 3tpsp olive oil

- One chopped shallot

- One chopped bulb fennel

- 2 oz. cheese

DIRECTIONS

1. In a bowl, whisk cream and egg till the mixture becomes smooth.

2. Take a skillet and heat it, then adds oil and heat for 1 minute.

3. Add shallots, fennel, and salt and cook for 4 min.

4. Add trout and tomatoes and cook for 1 min.

5. Bring the cooked egg up by scraping the pan bottom with a spatula.

6. Repeat it twice.

7. Sprinkle basil and cheese on top.

8. Broil the frittata in the preheated broiler for 4 to 5 min.

9. Cool and serve it.

NUTRITION: Calories: 190 cal Fat: 13 g Protein: 15 g Carbs: 1.5 g

6. Sausage and Peppers

Ready in: 60 minutes

Servings: 6

Difficulty: Medium

INGREDIENTS

- ¼ cup diced basil

- 3tbsp olive oil

- Salt as required

- Three bell peppers

- 1tbsp vinegar

- Pepper to taste

- Two minced garlic cloves

- Six sliced sausages

- 2tbsp oregano, dried

- One sliced onion

- 1tbsp red pepper, crushed

DIRECTIONS

10. Whisk red pepper, oil, oregano, vinegar, and garlic in a bowl.

11. Add onions and peppers in a bowl and top with sausages.

12. Bake it in preheated oven for 45 mins at 400°.

13. Top it with basil and enjoy.

NUTRITION: Calories: 208.3 cal Fat: 9.2 g Protein: 17.7 g Carbs: 12.5 g

7. Cheese and Sausage Breakfast

Ready in: 15 minutes

Servings: 4

Difficulty: Easy

INGREDIENTS

- Six eggs
- ¾ cup cheese, shredded
- ¾ cup milk
- Six pork sausage

DIRECTIONS

1. Deep fry sausages in the pan over medium flame.
2. Slice them into small pieces.
3. Whisk milk and eggs in a bowl.
4. Take a skillet and pour eggs in it, then add cheese and cook.
5. When eggs are cooked, stir them in sausage.
6. Serve and enjoy.

NUTRITION: Calories: 313 cal Fat: 23.2 g Protein: 22.5 g Carbs: 3 g

8. Creamy Zucchini

Ready in: 20 minutes

Servings: 6

Difficulty: Easy

INGREDIENTS

- Cheese, shredded

- 1 ½ tsp garlic, minced

- Four chopped zucchini

- 6 oz. cubed cream cheese

- 1/8 tsp pepper, ground

- 2tbsp olive oil

- ¼ tsp salt

- Nutmeg, ground

- 1 cup cream

DIRECTIONS

1. Sauté zucchini in a pan for 4-5 mins.

2. Add garlic in it and cook for a minute.

3. Now drain zucchini from the pan.

4. In the same pan, add cream and cream cheese cook over low flame.

5. Add zucchini mixture into this pan and cook with stirring.

6. Sprinkle it with nutmeg, pepper, and salt.

7. Serve and enjoy.

NUTRITION: Calories: 211.6 cal Fat: 18.9 g Protein: 4.4 g Carbs: 7.6 g

9. Kale and Cheese

Ready in: 15 minutes

Servings: 8

Difficulty: Easy

INGREDIENTS

- 2 cups Cheddar cheese, shredded

- Two bunch of kale

DIRECTIONS

1. Wash and dry kale and dice it into thin slices.

2. Spray cooking oil on baking sheets.

3. Spread kale over baking sheets and top it with cheddar cheese.

4. Bake it in the preheated oven at 425 F for 10-12 mins.

5. Serve and enjoy.

NUTRITION: Calories: 170 cal Fat: 10.1 g Protein: 10.7 g Carbs: 11.6 g

10. Tomato Quiche

Ready in: 1 hour 10 minutes

Servings: 8

Difficulty: Difficult

INGREDIENTS

- 1 ½ cup cream

- Dough

- Four eggs

- 1 cup onion, chopped

- 2 cups cheese

- 1 tsp salt

- 2tbsp butter

- ¼ tsp thyme, dried

- Four chopped tomatoes

- ¼ tsp pepper

DIRECTIONS

1. Roll the dough and transfer it to the baking dish as a crust.

2. Sauté onions in a pan over medium flame and thyme, salt, tomatoes, and pepper in it.

3. Cook it for 10-12 mins over medium flame.

4. In a baking dish, add cheese and top it with tomatoes and sprinkle the remaining cheese.

5. Beat eggs in a separate bowl and pour it.

6. Bake it in the preheated oven at 425 Fahrenheit for 10-12 mins.

7. Reduce the heat of the oven to 325 Fahrenheit and bake it for 40 mins.

NUTRITION: Calories: 484 cal Fat: 35 g Protein: 15 g Carbs: 7 g

11. Salmon Quiche

Ready in: 1 hour 10 minutes

Servings: 8

Difficulty: difficult

INGREDIENTS

- 1tbsp butter

- ¼ tsp salt

- One pastry shell, unbaked

- 2 cups cream

- One chopped onion

- Five eggs

- 2 cups cheese, shredded

- Parsley

- One can salmon

DIRECTIONS

1. In a pan, add butter and sauté onions in it.

2. Add cheese to the crust and then top t with onion and salmon.

3. Whisk salt, cream, and onion in a bowl and pour it over the salmon mixture.

4. Now, bake it for 50 mins at 350 Fahrenheit.

5. Serve and enjoy.

NUTRITION (per slice): Calories: 448 cal Fat: 29 g Protein: 26 g Carbs: 18 g

Chapter 2: Lunch Recipes

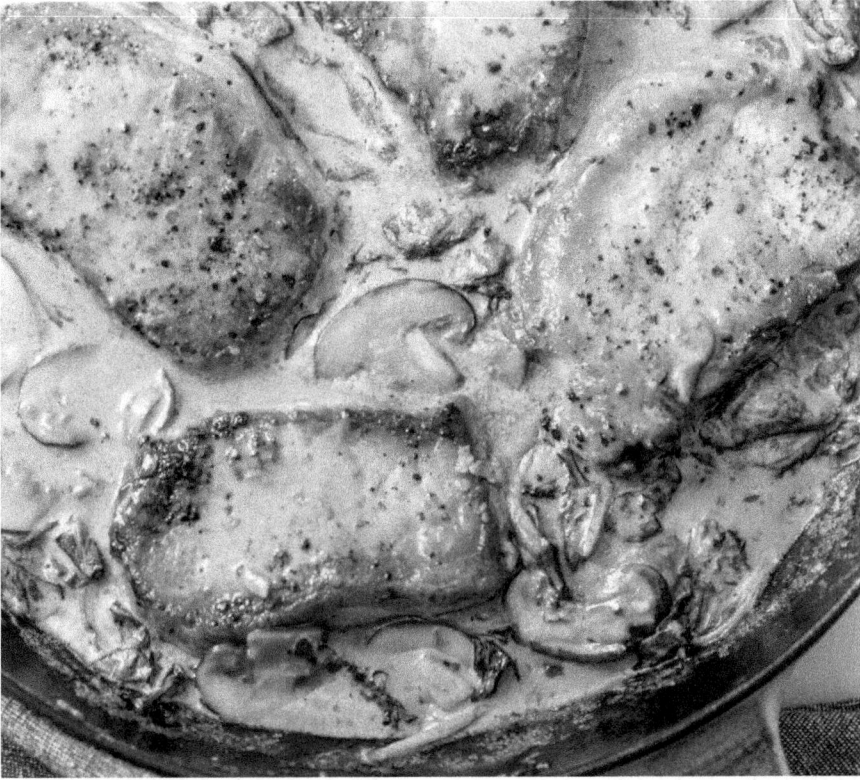

1. Lamb Meatballs

Ready in: 50 minutes

Servings: 4

Difficulty: medium

INGREDIENTS

- One egg, chopper

- 1 lb lamb

- 2 tbsp crushed parsley

- Three bulbs chopped garlic.

- 1 tsp cumin

- 2 tsp crushed oregano

- ½ tsp black pepper

- 1 tsp salt

- 3 tbsp olive oil

- ¼ tsp red chili powder

Green Goddess sauce

- 1 ½ cup basil

- 1 ½ cup Yogurt

- ½ cup mayonnaise

- ¼ crushed chives

- ½ parsley

- 1 tbsp lemon juice

- ¼ cup oregano

- Black pepper to taste

- Two bulb garlic

- Salt to taste

DIRECTIONS

1. Preheat the oven to 425 Fahrenheit. Using parchment paper, cover a large baking sheet. Combine all the ingredients except for sauce in a bowl.

2. Make meatballs out of the batter.

3. Drizzle oil and bake for 20 mins.

4. In the meantime, whisk the ingredients of the sauce in a bowl and blend.

5. Serve the meatballs warm with a dipping sauce made from the green goddess.

NUTRITION: Calories: 670 kcal Fat: 198 g Protein: 48 g Carbs: 67 g

2. Lamb Chops with Garlic Mint Sauce

Ready in: 21 minutes

Servings: 4

Difficulty: Easy

INGREDIENTS

- ½ tsp salt

- 3 lb slice Lamb

- ½ tsp black pepper

- 2 tbsp olive oil

- Mint and Garlic sauce

- 1 tbsp vinegar

- Three bulbs garlic

- 1 tbsp sesame oil

- 2 tbsp soy sauce

- 2 tbsp crushed mint

- ½ tsp red pepper

DIRECTIONS

1. Ready the barbecue and the lamb: Preheat the grill pan over high heat until nearly smoking. All sides of the lamb chops should be seasoned with salt and pepper.

2. Make the sauce: In a mixing cup, whisk together all of the sauce ingredients.

3. Barbecue: Coat or clean the grill pan with cooking spray or olive oil. Sear the chops for 2 mins in a hot grill pan, then flip them and heat for 3 1/2 mins on med or 2 1/2 mins on med-rare.

4. To eat, drizzle a generous amount of garlic and mint sauce over each chop.

NUTRITION: Calories: 482 kcal Fat: 26 g Protein: 5 g Carbs: 2 g

3. Potato and Beet Hash with Poached Eggs and Greens

Ready in: 45 minutes

Servings: 5

Difficulty: Easy

INGREDIENTS

- 2 cups chopped gold potato

- 2 tbsp olive oil

- 1 cup crushed onion

- 1 tbsp crushed sage

- 2 cups chopped sweet potato

- One cup cooked red beets.

- Three bulbs chopped garlic

- ½ tsp black pepper

- ½ tsp salt

- Four eggs

- 5 tsp wine vinegar

- 6 cups radicchio

- ½ tsp mustard

DIRECTIONS

1. Heat on med heat 1 tbsp oil in a large nonstick skillet. Add the onion to the skillet and roast for 5 mins, or till golden brown and tender. Cook, stirring regularly, for 25 mins or until potatoes are soft, adding two tsp sage and garlic as desired. Cook for 10 mins, stirring regularly, after adding the beets, 1/4 tsp salt, and 1/4 tsp pepper.

2. Fill a large skillet two-thirds full of water. Reduce to low heat after bringing to boil and proceed to cook. One tbsp of vinegar Each egg should be split into a custard cup and carefully poured into the pan. Cook for 3 mins, or until cooked to your taste. Using a slotted spoon, scrape the eggs from the pan. Evenly scatter 1/2 tsp sage over eggs.

3. Inside a large mixing bowl, beat together the remaining 1 tbsp oil, 2 tsp vinegar, 1/4 tsp salt, 1/2 tsp sage, 1/4 tsp pepper, and mustard. Toss in the frisée to coat. Serve with eggs and hash.

NUTRITION: Calories: 329 kcal Fat: 11.5 g Protein: 11.7 g Carbs: 45.5 g

4. Moroccan Lamb

Ready in: 45 minutes

Servings: 4

Difficulty: Medium

INGREDIENTS

- 3 tsp cinnamon

- 500g lamb

- 2 tsp paprika

- Olive oil

- Two tomatoes, sliced

- 1 tbsp crushed parsley

- ½ tsp chopped garlic

DIRECTIONS

1. Inside a large frying pan, heat the oil. Cook the lamb completely on both sides without using any additional oil. Add the spices and simmer for another min or until fragrant.

2. Bring the tomatoes and parsley to a boil, then reduce to low heat and roast for 30 mins, or till your lamb is tender. Serve with more parsley on top.

NUTRITION: Calories:350 kcal Fat: 22 g Protein: 27 g Carbs: 13 g

5. Paleo Lamb Meatloaf

Ready in: 110 minutes

Servings: 6

Difficulty: Difficult

INGREDIENTS

- ½ chopped onion

- 2 tbsp olive oil

- Salt to taste

- Two chopped celery ribs

- One ¼ lb lamb

- ½ tsp chili

- ½ cup coconut flour

- Two chopped eggs

- ½ tsp parsley

- 1/3 cup tomato ketchup

- ½ tsp rosemary

- ½ tsp basil

- 1 tsp cumin

- ½ tsp thyme

- ½ cup goat feta

- 2 tsp coconut sauce

DIRECTIONS

1. Preheat the oven to 400 Fahrenheit. Using parchment paper, baking pan such that it stretches over the sides and forms handles.

2. In a med sautés pan, heat the olive oil over med-low heat. Cook, occasionally stirring, until the onions and celery are soft for about 10-15 mins.

3. Combine all the remaining ingredients and stir well. Mix thoroughly. Fill baking tray halfway with the batter. Ketchup can be spread on top.

4. Place the baking pan inside and Preheat the oven. To prevent the top from cracking, place a pan of hot water on the oven rack below the meatloaf pan. Preheat the oven and bake for one hour.

5. Serve and enjoy it.

NUTRITION: Calories: 215 kcal Fat: 14 g Protein: 17 g Carbs: 5 g

6. Beef & Walnut Stir Fry with Veggie Rice

Ready in: 20 minutes

Servings: 2

Difficulty: Easy

INGREDIENTS

- One red chili powder

- 1 tbsp coconut oil

- 2 tsp honey

- Two steaks, slice

- 3 tbsp walnuts, toast

- Three sliced onion

- 2 tsp coconut oil

- ½ cup basil

- Six broccoli cut into pieces

- Four cauliflower cut into pieces.

- Black pepper to taste.

- ½ lemon juice

- Salt to taste

DIRECTIONS

1. In a wok, until hot, heat half of the oil.

2. Cook for 2-3 mins with the pepper before withdrawing from the wok.

3. Fried for 3 mins the beef in the remaining oil, then the peppers, spring onions, & walnuts, along with soy or tamari sauce & honey is added.

4. Cook for 1 min, stirring well.

5. Season to taste with pepper and salt before mixing in the basil leaves just before eating.

6. Blitz the cauliflower and broccoli until they are finely chopped.

7. Heat the coconut oil in a large skillet, and cook the vegetables for 5 mins, stirring continuously.

8. Only before serving the beef, season it and add the lemon zest and juice.

NUTRITION: Calories: 731 kcal Fat: 25 g Protein: 51 g Carbs: 17 g

7. Loaded Lebanese Rice: Yahweh

Ready in: 50 minutes

Servings: 5

Difficulty: Easy

INGREDIENTS

- Olive oil

- 1 ½ cups Grain rice

- 1 lb. beef

- One sliced onion

- ½ tsp garlic paste.

- One ¾ tsp allspice

- Pepper to taste

- ¾ tsp cinnamon

- ¾ ground cloves

- Salt to taste

- ½ cup pine

- ½ cup sliced parsley

- ½ cup raisins

- ½ cup almonds

DIRECTIONS

1. Soak the rice in chilly water for 15 mins.

2. In a pot, heat oil. Add cleaved red onions, cook on med-high warmth momentarily; at that point, the ground beef is added. Season the mixture of meat with allspice (one ¼ tsp), minced garlic, ground cloves (½ tsp), ground cinnamon (½ tsp), salt, & pepper. Cook until the meat is completely caramelized (8-10 mins).

3. Top the meat with rice. The rice is seasoned with salt and the rest of the allspice, cinnamon, and ground cloves. Add one tbsp of olive oil to cover the rice and 2 ½ cups of water.

4. Turn warmth to high and carry the fluid to a moving bubble. Let bubble until the fluid has fundamentally diminished (see picture beneath).

5. Now go warmth to low and cover; let cook for 20 mins or until dampness has been ingested and the rice is not. Remove from warmth and put in a safe spot for 10 mins.

6. Uncover the rice pot and spot an enormous round serving platter on the launch of the rice pot. Cautiously the pot substance is flipped on the platter.

7. Garnish with almonds, toasted pine nuts, raisins, and parsley.

NUTRITION: Calories: 389 kcal Fat: 30.9 g Protein: 20.1 g Carbs: 11.1 g

8. Corned Beef & Cauli Hash

Ready in: 30 minutes

Servings: 4

Difficulty: Easy

INGREDIENTS

- 3 cups of cooked corned beef

- One head of chopped fresh cauliflower

- 1/2 yellow onion, chopped

- 1 tbsp olive oil

- salt and pepper

- 1 tsp Cajun seasoning

- Optional: 4 eggs

- Garnish: Fresh chopped parsley

DIRECTIONS

1. Take a medium-sized skillet and heat olive oil in it.

2. Take water in a bowl and put some chopped cauliflower.

3. Put the bowl in the microwave for 3-5 minutes.

4. Take a skillet and brown the onion in it over medium flame.

5. Add 2-3 tbsp of water.

6. Once cauliflower is steamed, let it set for some time.

7. Mix the cauliflower and seasonings in skillet and mix.

8. Now add the beef and cook for 3-5 minutes.

9. Put some salt and pepper according to taste and garnish with parsley and top with eggs.

10. Serve and enjoy.

NUTRITION: Calories: 221 Cal Fat: 14 g Protein: 23 g Carbs: 2 g

9. Baked Sea Bass with Pesto, Zucchini, and Carrots

Ready in: 25-35 minutes

Servings: 4

Difficulty: Easy

INGREDIENTS

- 3/4 tsp salt

- Four sea-bass fillets, about 1 inch thick

- 1/2 tsp fresh-ground black pepper

- 1/4 cup of pesto, store-bought/homemade

- Three carrots, grated

- One zucchini, grated

- 2 tbsps olive oil

- 1/4 cup of dry white wine

DIRECTIONS

1. Take a baking dish, place Al-foil over it, and heat the microwave to 400.

2. Rub fish with pepper and salt.

3. Spread it with pesto. Cover it with carrots and top with zucchini. Gather around the foil and drizzle with olive oil. Make a sealed package and put it on the baking sheet.

4. Bake it for 10-15 minutes. Open the package and transfer them to the plates.

5. Enjoy.

NUTRITION: Calories: 265 Cal Fat: 10 g Protein: 34 g Carbs: 9 g

10. Sriracha Tuna Chili

Ready in: 20 minutes

Servings: 5

Difficulty: Easy

INGREDIENTS

- 2 Tbsps Canola Oil

- 2 cups of Tuna

- 15 oz fried Vegetables

- 16 oz Kidney Beans

- 1.25 oz Chili Seasoning

- 15 oz Beans

- 10 Tbsps Salsa

- 10 Tsp Chili Sauce

- 50g Sriracha

- 28 oz Crushed Tomatoes

- 2 Tsp Garlic

DIRECTIONS

1. Take beans in a bowl and rinse well.

2. Drain the tuna.

3. Take a pan and heat olive oil on a medium flame.

4. Once the pan is heated, add the remaining ingredients to it and mix well.

5. Cook for 15-20 minutes and keep moving with a spatula after regular intervals.

6. Serve and enjoy.

NUTRITION: Calories: 380 Cal Fat: 6 g Protein: 32 g Carbs: 49.5 g

11. Poached Cod with Tomato and Saffron

Ready in: 10-15 minutes

Servings: 4

Difficulty: Easy

INGREDIENTS

- 2 tbsps olive oil

- Two mashed garlic cloves

- 1 tsp crushed pepper

- 14.5-oz tomatoes

- 1/4 cup of wine

- Two bay leaves

- Saffron threads Pinch

- Kosher salt, freshly ground pepper

- 4 oz skinless cod fillets

DIRECTIONS

1. Take a skillet and heat olive oil over medium flame.

2. Add garlic & Aleppo pepper to it. Cook for 3-5 minutes.

3. Crush the tomatoes with hands and add with bay leaves and a 1-4th cup of water. Cook it and bring a boil.

4. Season with salt and pepper.

5. Transfer cod to bowls and spoon with the poaching liquid.

7. Enjoy.

NUTRITION: Calories: 429 Cal Fat: 15 g Protein: 37 g Carbs: 38 g

12. Garlic Parmesan Roasted Radishes

Ready in: 50 minutes

Servings: 4

Difficulty: Easy

INGREDIENTS

- 2 tsp chopped rosemary

- Two bundle radishes

- Four bulbs chopped garlic

- Two olive oil

- 2 tbsp butter

- ¼ cup cheese

- Salt to taste

DIRECTIONS

1. Up to 400 Fahrenheit, preheat the oven and cover a baking sheet with parchment paper.

2. Combine radishes, melted butter, minced garlic, rosemary, cinnamon, and pepper in a mixing bowl. Toss all together thoroughly. 45 mins of roasting

3. Coat all of the radishes with parmesan cheese. Cook for another 5 mins, or until golden and crisp.

4. When finished, serve the roasted radishes as a side dish or as a full meal.

NUTRITION: Calories: 87 kcal Fat: 7 g Protein: 2 g Carbs: 2 g

13. Balsamic Roasted Cabbage Steaks

Ready in: 40minutes

Servings: 6

Difficulty: Medium

INGREDIENTS

- ½ tsp mustard

- ¼ cup olive oil

- 2 tbsp vinegar

- ½ tsp honey

- One bulb chopped garlic

- Parsley as required

- Salt to taste

- Black pepper to taste

DIRECTIONS

1. Preheat the oven to 400 Fahrenheit.

2. Gently oil a baking sheet and set it aside.

3. Cut the cabbage's bottom (root) and set it up on the cutting board with the flat end facing up; slice into 1-inch thick slices.

4. Place cabbage slices on a baking sheet that has already been prepared.

5. In a mixing cup, add the extra virgin olive oil, balsamic vinegar, mustard, garlic, sugar, salt, and pepper.

6. Spray all sides of the cabbage steaks with the prepared balsamic glaze.

7. Roast for 20 to 25 mins, or until the potatoes are crispy and tender.

NUTRITION: Calories: 87 kcal Fat: 9 g Protein: 0.5 g Carbs: 1 g

14. Grilled eggplant, tomato, and Mint Salad

Ready in: 40 minutes

Servings: 4

Difficulty: Medium

INGREDIENTS

- Salt to taste

- Two eggplants cut into a piece.

- Olive oil as required

- Black pepper to taste

- 2 tbsp lemon juice

- One bulb chopped garlic

- 1 tbsp sugar

- 1 tbsp red chili

- ¼ cup crushed mint

- 6 tbsp olive oil

- ½ grape tomatoes

- ½ cup crushed parsley

DIRECTIONS

1. Salt the eggplant generously and spread it out on a towel-lined baking sheet in a single layer. After 30 mins, blot the eggplant dry and spray generously with olive oil on both sides; set aside.

2. In a chimney starter, light 6 quarts of charcoal and heat until the coals are filled with a fine grey ash coating, about 15 mins. Cover half of the barbecue with charcoal, cover with the grill grate, and heat for 5 mins. Clean the grate with a scraper.

3. Grill eggplant for 2-4 mins, or until browned. Cook for another 3 mins until the eggplant is finely browned and tender.

4. To make the emulsion, mix the garlic, cayenne, lemon juice, pepper, sugar, a pinch of salt, and 6 tbsps olive oil.

5. Cut eggplant to make it half-inch-wide strips, and with dressing, toss it.

NUTRITION: Calories: 310 kcal Fat: 27.6 g Protein: 2.9 g Carbs:16.3 g

Chapter 3: Dinner Recipes

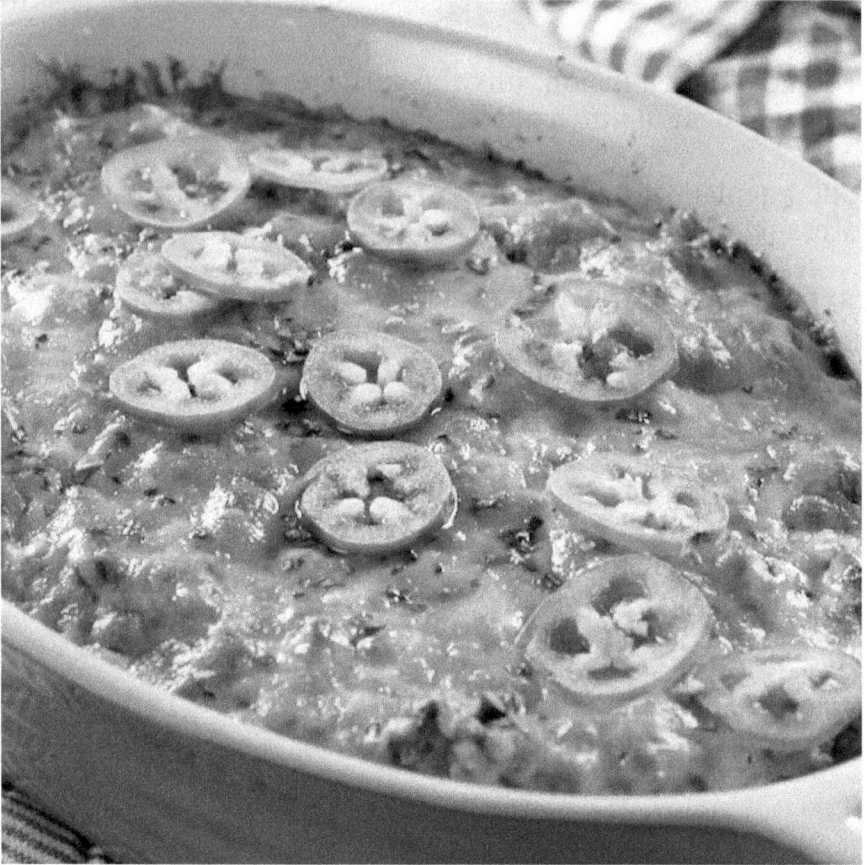

1. Cajun Crabmeat Casserole

Ready in: 65 minutes

Servings: 6

Difficulty: Medium

INGREDIENTS

- 2 ½ tbsp butter

- 1/3 cup crushed celery

- 1/3 cups sliced scallion

- ½ cup green chili paste

- 6 tbsp mayonnaise

- Two cloves garlic paste

- 1 tbsp mustard

- 2 tsp sauce

- 2 tsp crushed parsley

- Salt to taste

- 1 tsp tabasco sauce

- 1 tsp cayenne pepper

- One egg

- 1 cup cream

- 1 lb lump crabmeat

- Paprika to taste

DIRECTIONS

1. Add butter to a saucepan and melt it at medium heat. Add celery, garlic, scallions, and bell pepper in it and cook it for a time until vegetables are tender.

2. Take the pan from heat and add other ingredients like mustard, mayonnaise, parsley, Worcestershire sauce, salt, cayenne, and Tabasco and stir them until completely blended.

3. Add this mixture to the egg and mix them smoothly.

4. Now add crabmeat and pour this mixture into the casserole dish.

5. Drizzle cream throughout the mixture

6. Place this mixture in the oven that is already heated at 350°F and bake it for 20 minutes.

7. Serve immediately.

NUTRITION: Calories: 450 kcal Fat: 51 g Protein: 20 g Carbs: 31 g

2. Tuna Cauliflower Rice

Ready in: 15 minutes

Servings: 5

Difficulty: Easy

INGREDIENTS

- 1 tbsp coconut oil

- 2 tsp chopped Ginger

- One cloves crushed garlic

- 1 /4 cauliflower cut into slice

- Two crushed onion

- 1 cup chopped capsicum

- One crushed chili

- 2 tbsp coconut

- 2 tbsp crushed coriander

- 3 lb tuna

- 1 tbsp soy sauce

- 1 tbsp lemon juice

DIRECTIONS

1. Make a cauliflower recipe, make its small florets and then process it in a food processor, converting it into fine rice.

2. Take a frying pan, add olive oil to it, and heat it. Then add other ingredients like cauliflower, capsicum, garlic, ginger, chili, spring onions.

3. Now cook it for 1-2 minutes.

4. Now add tuna, coconut, and fresh lemon juice and cook it.

5. To make it tasty, season it with tamari. Serve it while hot.

NUTRITION: Calories: 108 kcal Fat: 3 g Protein: 7 g Carbs: 9 g

3. Crawfish Boil Recipe

Ready in: 60 minutes

Servings: 5

Difficulty: Medium

INGREDIENTS

- 3 lb crawfish

- 6 oz crawfish shrimp

- 10 cups water

- 2 tbsp Cajun seasoning

- One clove garlic

- 14 oz sausage

- 1 tbsp Lemon Pepper seasoning

- One minced lemon

- Three ears corn

- 13 oz chopped red potatoes

DIRECTIONS

1. Boil water in a pot.

2. Mix in seasoning, crab, lemon pepper, and shrimp and let it cook.

3. Stir in the potatoes, garlic, sausage, corn, and lemon slices. Cover and let it cook for 10 minutes.

4. Transfer the crawfish into the pot and cook for 3-4 minutes, with the lid covered.

5. Turn off the heat and let the crawfish soak for 10 minutes.

6. Remove all the ingredients using a strainer and serve immediately. Discard the crawfish boil water.

NUTRITION: Calories: 317 kcal Fat: 18 g Protein: 16 g Carbs: 22 g

4. Thai Coconut Clams

Ready in: 30 minutes

Servings: 5

Difficulty: Easy

INGREDIENTS

- One lemon cut into slices

- 1 tbsp coconut oil

- One stalk lemongrass

- Three chopped shallots

- ½ cup vegetable soup

- Two jalapeno peppers

- 1 tbsp chopped ginger

- 2 tbsp sauce

- ½ cup coconut milk

- 1 tbsp sugar

- 2 lb scrubbed

- One crushed scallion

- Salt to taste

- ½ cup crushed cilantro leaves

DIRECTIONS

1. For this recipe, take a pressure cooker, add oil to it and boil it. Then add sauté and shallots and cook for 3-5 minutes until they become soft and brown at the edges.

2. While cooking, take a lemongrass stalk and remove its outer layers and bruise its core.

3. Take the instant pot and add ginger, jalapeños, fish sauce, brown sugar, and lemongrass stalk. Continuously stir it and make sure that brown sugar is completely dissolved. Then add coconut milk and stir it again for 5 minutes and simmer.

4. Finally, add clams and cook it at low heat for 1-2 minutes. If any claim is not open, remove it. Taste it and add pepper and salt to make it tastier.

5. Serve clams in bowls.

NUTRITION: Calories: 233 kcal Fat: 10 g Protein: 12.5 g Carbs: 18 g

5. Lobster Chili

Ready in: 35 minutes

Servings: 5

Difficulty: Medium

INGREDIENTS

- 2 ½ lb meat

- Six chopped bacon

- Four cloves chopped garlic

- Two chopped onion

- Two crushed jalapeno pepper

- 3 tbsp red chili

- 2 cups kidney beans

- 6 cup tomatoes paste

- 1 tsp cumin

- Salt to taste

- 1 tsp wine vinegar

- 4 oz green chili

DIRECTIONS

1. Take a pot or an oven and add bacon to it and cook at low to medium heat.

2. Use a slotted spoon to remove bacon from the pot and reserve it while leaving bacon fat in the pot. Do not remove bacon fat.

3. Now add sliced onions in bacon fat and cook it for 3-4 minutes at low heat. or when you notice it has become soft.

4. Now add garlic, chili powder, and jalapeños, stir them and cook for 5-10 minutes.

5. Then add tomatoes, vinegar, beans, cumin oregano, and salt, similarly stir them as well.

6. Cook this mixture for up to 20-30 minutes or when it becomes thicken. Liquid smoke can also be added to give it a smoky flavor.

7. Now it is time to add reserved bacon, Maine Lobster, and green chile. Simmer it for few minutes.

NUTRITION: Calories: 419 kcal Fat: 13.5 g Protein: 7 g Carbs: 50.2 g

6. Lobster Deviled Eggs

Ready in: 68 minutes

Servings: 24

Difficulty: Medium

INGREDIENTS

- 1 tbsp paprika

- 12 eggs, cooked

- 1 ½ tsp mustard

- Crushed chives

- ¾ cup mayonnaise

- ½ tsp black pepper

- Red pepper to taste

- Salt to taste

- 1 cup crushed lobster, cooked

DIRECTIONS

1. To make lobster deviled eggs main ingredients are needed eggs and lobsters. First, using a knife lengthwise, cut the eggs. Take one bowl and a serving plate. Pour egg yolk in the bowl while egg white in the serving plate. Using a fork, mash egg yolk and add mayonnaise to it. Using a mixer, mix them smoothly. Then add lobster and stir

2. On the top of egg white, spray paprika and chives, cover it, and place it in a freezer. When it is chilled, it is ready to serve.

NUTRITION: Calories: 141 kcal Fat: 11 g Protein: 7 g Carbs: 2 g

7. Steamed Clams in Spicy Tomato Sauce

Ready in: 60 minutes

Servings: 4

Difficulty: Medium

INGREDIENTS

- 1 tsp orange juice

- 4 ½ lb clams

- 1 cup wine

- 2 tbsp olive oil

- One chopped onion

- 28 oz tomatoes juice

- ¼ red chili

- ¼ tsp sugar

- Saffron to taste

- 1 tsp thyme

- Salt to taste

- Olive oil

- 4 tbsp crushed parsley

- Lemon juice

DIRECTIONS

1. Clean the clams with a tiny tool, such as a toothbrush, after rinsing them in many changes of water. Anything that is accessible or has broken shells should be discarded.

1. Spoon the wine into a wide, lidded pan large enough to contain each of the clams. Take to the boil, then minimize to half the original number. Add some clams, cover, and cook for 2-3 mins on high heat, tossing the pan periodically before the clams open. Switch off the sun. Some claims that haven't opened can be discarded.

2. Wash the clams in a strainer onto a container lined with cheesecloth. In different cups, put aside the liquid & the clams. Hold your clams in their shells or cut them, whatever is more practical for serving.

3. In a big, broad, lidded skillet or casserole, heat the olive oil on medium heat & add the shallots. Cook for 3 minutes, stirring regularly, until the vegetables are soft, then incorporate the garlic & red pepper flakes. Cook, stirring continuously for 30

secs to 1 min until it is fragrant, then add the tomatoes with juice, thyme, orange zest, saffron, sugar, and clam liquid. Season with salt & pepper to taste, then bring to a boil over medium heat for 20-25 mins, stirring regularly, until the mixture has thoroughly cooked & is very fragrant. Season with salt and pepper to taste.

4. Heat the clams in the tomato sauce, stirring continuously. Stir in parsley or cilantro and serve in big soup cups. Drizzle each serving with some olive oil and several drops of lemon juice.

NUTRITION: Calories: 602 kcal Fat: 12 g Protein: 77 g Carbs: 32 g

8. Smoked Cod Pate Platter

Ready in: 15 minutes

Servings: 5

Difficulty: Easy

INGREDIENTS

- 3 tbsp Yoghurt

- Two smoked Cod Fillets

- ½ tbsp lemon juice

To Serve

- Apple coleslaw

- Eight oatcakes

- Four chopped radishes

- Four celery sticks

- Four artichoke

Apple coleslaw

- 100 g chopped cabbage

- 100 ml crème

- One lemon juice

- 1 tsp mustard

- 100 g chopped fennel

- One chopped carrot

DIRECTIONS

1. Take a mixing bowl, add cod in it and mesh it smoothly. Then add yogurt, black pepper, and lemon juice. Using a mixer mesh these ingredients as well as make a chunky paste. Pour this mixture into a serving bowl, and it is ready to serve.

2. This chunky pate can be served along with coleslaw and other ingredients on the serving plate.

3. To prepare coleslaw using a mixer, make a mixture of lemon juice, crème Fraiche, and mustard. Also, add vegetables and fruits like apples.

NUTRITION: Calories: 331 kcal Fat: 12 g Protein: 52 g Carbs: 1 g

9. Herbed Cherry Tomatoes

Ready in: 10 minutes

Servings: 4

Difficulty: Easy

INGREDIENTS

- ½ tsp sugar

- 4 cups cherry tomatoes

- 3 tbsp vinegar

- ¼ cup oil

- ¼ cup minced parsley

- 1 ½ tsp chopped oregano

- 1 ½ tsp chopped basil

- ½ tsp salt

DIRECTIONS

1. Take a bowl, add tomatoes to it, and add salt, pepper and vinegar, basil, oregano, and parsley. Add the tomatoes to it.

2. Serve with lettuce leaves.

NUTRITION: Calories: 56 cal Fat: 5 g Protein: 1 g Carbs: 4 g

10. Garlic Seasoned Vegetable Spinach Russian salad

Ready in: 35 minutes

Servings: 6

Difficulty: Easy

INGREDIENTS

- Two minced garlic clove

- One ¾ cups chicken stock

- 4 cups chopped vegetables

DIRECTIONS

1. Take a pan, add the broth, vegetables, and garlic, cook it until the vegetables get soft and broth get a boil, add the salt and pepper according to taste.

2. Strain the water from the vegetables and serve.

NUTRITION: Calories: 208 cal Fat: 18.3 g Protein: 2.7 g Carbs: 9.8 g

11. Savoy Cabbage with Pine Nuts and Sesame Seeds

Ready in: 25 minutes

Servings: 4

Difficulty: Easy

INGREDIENTS

- 3 tbsp balsamic vinegar

- One savoy cabbage

- One onion

- Salt to taste

- 3 tbsp sesame seeds

- 4 tbsp olive oil

- 3 tbsp pine nuts

- Black pepper to taste

DIRECTIONS

1. Slice the cabbage. Take a pan, boil water with some salt, add the cabbage to it, and blanch.

2. Take onions and dice them into rings, sauté them in the oil with some pinenuts and cook for about 5 minutes. Add the cabbage, pepper, and salt.

3. Drizzle vinegar and garnish it with onions.

4. Serve and enjoy it.

NUTRITION: Calories: 126 kcal Fat: 7 g Protein: 5 g Carbs: 15 g

12. Stuffed Cabbage with Ricotta and Pine Nuts

Ready in: 50 minutes

Servings: 4

Difficulty: Medium

INGREDIENTS

- 1 ½ tbsp sugar

- 2 tbsp butter

- 1/8 cup rice

- 1 ½ oz noodles

- One ¼ cup water

- One cabbage

- Salt to taste

- 1/3 cup roasted pine nuts

- ¼ cup shredded cheese, parmesan

- ¾ cup ricotta

- 1 ½ cup vegetable stock

- 3 tbsp diced basil

- Three minced garlic cloves

- 4 tbsp diced parsley

- Black pepper to taste

DIRECTIONS

1. Take a pan, add butter in it, let it melt, add the pinenut, toss the nuts into the batter, and then add the rice and water. Let it simmer for 10-15 mins.

2. Cut the cabbage and blanch it in saltwater for 5 minutes, and then tap dry.

3. Add 2 tbsp cheese(parmesan), garlic, salt, pepper, basil, and parsley, toss them all. Add this nuts mixture to an ovenproof dish and add cabbage at the top of the nuts and rice mixture.

Pour the broth, salt, sugar, and pepper mixture at the top and bake it for 35 minutes until the liquid is evaporated.

NUTRITION: Calories: 963 cal Fat: 48 g Protein: 21 g Carbs: 114 g

13. Red Cabbage with Apple, Pinenuts, and Sultanas

Ready in: 30 minutes

Servings: 5

Difficulty: Easy

INGREDIENTS

- 2 tbsp lime juice

- 3 ½ cups diced cabbage

- One chopped apple

- ½ diced onion

- ¼ cup roasted pine nuts

- Two minced garlic cloves

- ¼ cup sultanas

- Salt to taste

DIRECTIONS

1. Take a large saucepan, add some oil, sauté cabbage, onion, garlic for 5-6 minutes in oil. Sprinkle pepper, salt, verjuice, and water; cook until the water evaporates, and the cabbage is softened.

2. Add the pine nuts sultanas and toss them all and cook for few minutes.

3. Serve and enjoy!

NUTRITION: Calories: 963 kcal Fat: 48 g Protein: 21 g Carbs: 114 g

14. Farfalle with Savoy Cabbage, Pancetta and Mozzarella

Ready in: 35 minutes

Servings: 5

Difficulty: Medium

INGREDIENTS

- 7 oz chopped cheese, mozzarella

- ¼ cup olive oil

- 3 tbsp pine nuts

- ¼ lb diced pancetta

- 2 tsp diced thyme

- One ¾ lb savory cabbage

- One chopped garlic clove

- ¼ cup shredded cheese, parmesan

- Salt to taste

- ½ cup water

- Pepper to taste

- 1 lb farfalle

DIRECTIONS

1. Take one large skillet, add oil and pancetta and fry it till golden. Sieve it and chopped it

2. Toast the pine nuts in a saucepan and put them on a plate now; in the skillet, add thyme and garlic, stir it and put some cabbage in it, sprinkle pepper, parmesan, salt, and some water, cook it on low heat

3. Boil some farfalle.

4. Add pasta in a pot, put the cabbage, season it with salt, parmesan pepper, pine nuts, pancetta, and leftover olive oil and stir it well till the cheese gets melted.

NUTRITION: Calories: 72 kcal Fat: 11 g Protein: 8 g Carbs: 2 g

15. Lemon, Black Pepper, Pecorino and Cabbage Rice

Ready in: 30 minutes

Servings: 4

Difficulty: Easy

INGREDIENTS

- 2 tbsp lemon juice

- Olive oil as required

- 1 ½ cups rice

- One diced onion

- ½ cup butter

- 1 tsp black pepper

- One ¼ quart boiling water

- ½ grated savoy cabbage

- 3 ½ oz shredded cheese, pecorino

DIRECTIONS

1. Take a large pan, and heat olive oil, sauté onions in the pan till it gets translucent

2. In a pot, add some butter and rice, stir it nicely, add water timely and don't try to turn the high flame stir it until the rice gets completely cooked

3. In rice, add sprinkle pepper, pecorino, lemon zest, and some butter to make it creamy.

4. Serve it warmly

NUTRITION: Calories: 131 kcal Fat: 6 g Protein: 5 g Carbs: 13 g

Chapter 4: Snacks Recipes

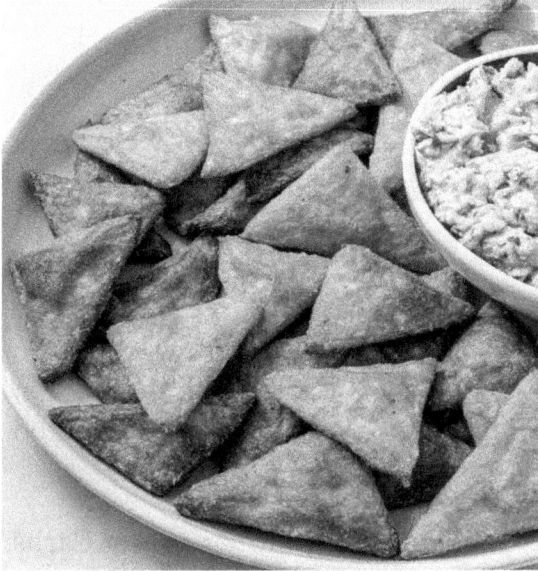

1. Kohl Slaw

Ready in: 75 minutes

Servings: 4

Difficulty: Medium

INGREDIENTS

- Four chopped carrots

- 2 tbsp vinegar

- 1 tbsp nectar

- Black pepper to taste

- 1 tbsp mayonnaise

- 1 tbsp mustard

- Two chopped apple

- Salt to taste

- Two chopped kohlrabi

DIRECTIONS

1. Combine mayonnaise, mustard, vinegar, Dijon, pepper, nectar & salt altogether in the bowl.

2. Mix apples, carrots & kohlrabi into dressing till finely coated. Cove & refrigerate for an hour.

NUTRITION: Calories: 138 kcal Fat: 2.6 g Protein: 3.2 g Carbs: 29.4 g

2. Cornbread Stuffing

Ready in: 60 minutes

Servings: 10

Difficulty: Medium

INGREDIENTS

- Black pepper to taste

- Two stick butter

- 2 tbsp chopped thyme

- 3 tbsp chopped sage

- 2 tbsp chopped parsley

- Salt to taste

- 1 tsp chopped rosemary

Stuffing

- ¾ cup milk

- Two chopped onion

- 9 cups sliced cornbread

- 1 cup chicken soup

- Three chopped celery stalks

- One beaten egg

DIRECTIONS

Cornbread

1. Preheat the oven to 300 Fahrenheit. Mix all the cornbread ingredients all together in a large bowl, then pour into the baking pan.

2. Bake it for 22-24mins / till its top becomes golden brown. Then set it aside to cool (almost overnight). Don't cover.

3. Preheat the oven to 250 Fahrenheit —slice cornbread into 1-inch cubes. You may have almost 7-8 cups cubes, then spread it on a lined baking sheet & bake for 10 min. Set it aside to cool while you'll prepare the stuffing. Set the oven up to 450 Fahrenheit.

Stuffing

1. Whisk broth & eggs in a bowl & set aside.

2. Heat the butter in a large pan on med-high heat. Now add onion, thyme celery, parsley, salt, sage, & pepper & cook for 4 mins till the vegetables begin to get soft. Then squeeze the sausage meat out of casings into the pan. Break it up using a spoon, then add pears & cook till sausage is recently cooked through. Now, pour into broth + egg mixture and any liquid present in the pan. Add toasted cornbread cubes & pecans. Now, gently fold everything all together.

3. Spoon the stuffing into a 9×13baking pan. Bake it for 40mins. Sprinkle it with more parsley (if you want) & serve warm.

NUTRITION: Calories: 354 kcal Fat: 16 g Protein: 14 g Carbs: 40 g

3. Roasted Pumpkin with Nuts and Manchego Cheese

Ready in: 35 minutes

Servings: 5

Difficulty: Easy

INGREDIENTS

- Black pepper to taste

- 2 lb pumpkins

- 2 oz parsley

- Salt to taste

- 3 tbsp olive oil

- ¾ cup hazelnuts

- 2 tsp slice thyme

- 2 tsp crushed Rosemary

- ½ lb cheese

DIRECTIONS

1. Preheat your oven to 400 Fahrenheit.

2. Slice pumpkin into wedges, almost 1" (2,5 cm) thick. You may peel off its skin using a sharp knife / just leave it & peel after it's serving.

3. Brush it with oil on both sides. Pepper & salt to taste. Now place them on the pan & bake it for 15mins / till the wedges of pumpkin get soft.

4. Chop those nuts roughly using a knife & mix with shredded manchego, chopped parsley, & rosemary / dried thyme.

5. Remove pumpkin from oven & spread herbs & nuts on the top & gratinate till cheese starts to melt.

6. Serve along with leafy greens & a splash of olive oil.

NUTRITION: Calories: 722 kcal Fat: 61 g Protein: 26 g Carbs: 18 g

4. Easy Hummus

Ready in: 10 minutes

Servings: 5

Difficulty: Easy

INGREDIENTS

- Paprika paste

- 15 oz chickpeas boiled

- ¼ cup sesame oil

- ¼ cup lemon juice

- 2 tbsp olive oil

- Salt to taste

- ½ tsp cumin

- 3 tbsp water

DIRECTIONS

1. Add all the ingredients in a food processor and blend to get a paste.

2. Transfer the paste in serving bowl.

3. Sprinkle olive oil and paprika and serve.

NUTRITION: Calories: 190 kcal Fat: 11 g Protein: 6 g Carbs: 18 g

5. Roasted Vegetables Tricolored

Ready in: 40 minutes

Servings: 5

Difficulty: Medium

INGREDIENTS

- ½ cup olive oil

- 1 lb Brussels

- 8 oz Mushroom

- 8 oz tomatoes

- Salt to taste

- 1 tsp crushed Rosemary

- ½ tsp black pepper

DIRECTIONS

1. To 200°C, preheat the oven. Rinse & trim all vegetables & peel the outer layer of the Brussels sprouts if needed.

2. Cut the vegetables so they're roughly the same size—place in a 9" baking dish.

3. Add spices & olive oil & mix.

4. Bake for 20 mins or till the vegetables have softened & turned a nice color.

5. Serve as a side dish with meat, chicken, or fish.

NUTRITION: Calories: 208 kcal Fat: 18 g Protein: 4 g Carbs: 6 g

6. Thai Curry Cabbage

Ready in: 30 minutes

Servings: 5

Difficulty: Easy

INGREDIENTS

- 1 tbsp sesame seeds oil

- 3 tbsp coconut oil

- 2 lb crushed cabbage

- 1 tbsp Thai red Curry

- Salt to taste

DIRECTIONS

1. Heat coconut oil in a wok over a high flame. Add curry paste & stir for a min. Add cabbage.

2. Sauté till the cabbage begins to turn golden brown, but still is a little chewy. Stir thoroughly & lower the heat towards the end.

3. Salt to taste. Add sesame oil & sauté for another 1–2 mins & serve.

NUTRITION: Calories: 181 kcal Fat: 13 g Protein: 3 g Carbs: 8 g

7. Pizza Fat Bombs

Ready in: 2 hours 45 minutes

Servings: 6

Difficulty: Difficult

INGREDIENTS

- 4 ounces of cream cheese softened

- ¼ cup of chopped pepperoni

- ¼ cup of chopped black olives

- 2 Tbsps chopped fresh basil

- 2 Tbsps shredded Parmesan cheese

- 2 Tbsps pizza sauce no-sugar-added

DIRECTIONS

1. preheat oven to 350 Fahrenheit. Line the baking sheet along with some parchment paper.

2. In a medium mixing cup, add all ingredients and pound on low speed with the handheld blender until completely mixed.

3. Chill for 30 minutes in the refrigerator.

5. Take out of the fridge & break into six equivalent parts. Make a ball out of each section and put it on the prepared baking sheet.

6. Chill for 2 hrs in the refrigerator. Switch to the airtight jar and hold refrigerated for up to one week before ready to feed.

NUTRITION: Calories: 131 Cal Fat: 10 g Protein: 3 g Carbs: 7 g

8. Swedish Meatballs

Ready in: 30 minutes

Servings: 5

Difficulty: Easy

INGREDIENTS

Meatballs

- 1/2 cup of breadcrumbs

- One large egg

- 1/2 cup of (125ml) milk

- 35 ml cream

- 1/3 tsp salt

- 1 tbsp garlic

- 1/4 tsp black pepper & ground white pepper each

- 1/4 tsp Grillkrydda / allspice / all-purpose seasoning

- 1/2 cup of finely chopped onion

- 1 lb. ground beef

- 1/2 lb. ground pork

- 2 tbsps finely chopped fresh parsley

- 2 tsp olive oil

- 1 tbsp butter

Gravy Sauce

- 1/3 cup of butter

- 1/4 cup of plain/all-purpose flour

- 250 ml beef broth (or stock)

- 250 ml vegetable broth

- 1 cup thickened cream

- 2 tsp soy sauce

- Salt & pepper

- 1 tsp Dijon mustard

DIRECTIONS

1. Combine the breadcrumbs, peppers, garlic, milk, egg, cinnamon, cream, and seasoning in a large mixing cup. Give at least 10 minutes for the milk to sink into the breadcrumbs.

2. Substitute the carrot, meat(s), & parsley after milk has consumed some of the oil. To blend, blend very well using your fingertips.

3. Shape the meat into roughly 24 tiny or 16 bigger balls.

4. In a medium-high-heat bowl, melt 1 tbsp of butter & 2 tsp of oil. To stop stewing or simmering, cook meatballs in two-batch batches. Wrap in foil and switch to the warm tray.

5. Melt the one-third cup butter in the skillet with the juices. Whisk throughout the flour till it's fully dissolved and brown in appearance. In a wide mixing cup, combine the broth, milk, soy sauce, and Dijon mustard. Season with pepper and salt to taste and carry to a boil. To blend both of the flavors, thoroughly combine the sauce.

7. Proceed to cook until the sauce has thickened.

NUTRITION: Calories: 484 Cal Fat: 41 g Protein: 18 g Carbs: 9 g

9. Scrambled Egg Wraps

Ready in: 20 minutes

Servings: 6

Difficulty: Easy

INGREDIENTS

- One chopped sweet red pepper

- One chopped green pepper

- 2 tsp canola oil

- Five plum tomatoes, seeded & chopped

- 1/2 cup of soy milk

- 1/4 tsp salt

- Six eggs

- Six tortillas

DIRECTIONS

1. Sauté peppers into the oil until soft in a broad nonstick skillet. Cook for the next 1 to 2 minutes after inserting the tomatoes. Whisk the soy milk, eggs, and salt together in a large mixing cup. Reduce the heat to mild and pour in the egg mixture. Cook, stirring continuously until the eggs are ready. Top each tortilla with 2/3 cup of the mixture and roll them up.

NUTRITION: Calories: 258 Cal Fat: 10 g Protein: 12 g Carbs: 30 g

10. Falafel

Ready in: 50 minutes

Servings: 1

Difficulty: Medium

INGREDIENTS

- 2 cups of dried chickpeas

- ½ tsp baking soda

- 1 cup parsley

- ¾ cup cilantro

- ½ cup dill

- One quartered small onion

- 7-8 peeled garlic cloves

- Salt

- 1 tbsp ground black pepper

- 1 tbsp ground cumin

- 1 tbsp ground coriander

- optional 1 tsp cayenne pepper

- 1 tsp baking powder

- 2 tbsp toasted sesame seeds

- Oil for frying

Falafel Sauce

- Tahini Sauce

Fixings for falafel sandwich (optional)

- Pita pockets

- Chopped or diced English cucumbers

- Tomatoes, chopped/diced

- Pickles

- Baby Arugula

DIRECTIONS

1. In a wide mixing cup, add both dried chickpeas & baking soda with sufficient water to cover the chickpeas by almost 2 inches. Soak for 18 hours overnight. When the chickpeas are finished, drain them full, then pat those dry.

2. In a wide bowl of the food processor equipped with a blade, mix the garlic, onions, herbs, chickpeas, and spices. Run the food processor for 40 seconds before all of the ingredients are well mixed and the falafel mixture is created.

3. Put that falafel mixture in a bowl and securely cover. Refrigerate for almost 1 hour (or up to one night) before cooking.

4. Add sesame seeds and baking powder to a falafel mixture well before frying and whisk with a spoon.

5. Scoop falafel mixture then shapes into 12-inch-thick patties. It's simpler to shape the patties with wet hands.

6. Dump 3 inches of oil into a medium saucepan. Heat this oil over medium to high heat until it gently bursts. Drop these falafel patties into the oil carefully and fry for 3-5 minutes, or until crispy and medium brown outside. If required, fry this falafel in batches to prevent crowding the plate.

8. Drain that fried-falafel patty in the colander or on a paper towel-lined pan.

9. Organize falafel patties into pita bread with tomato, hummus or tahini, arugula, and cucumbers, or assemble falafel patties into pita bread and hummus tahini, tomato, arugula, and cucumbers.

NUTRITION: Calories: 93 Cal Fat: 3.8 g Protein: 3.9 g Carbs: 1.4 g

11. Granola Bars

Ready in: 15 minutes

Servings: 2-4

Difficulty: Easy

INGREDIENTS

- One heaping cup of packed dates

- 1 1/2 cups of rolled oats

- 1/4 cup of creamy salted natural peanut butter /almond butter

- 1/4 cup of maple syrup /agave nectar

- 1 cup of roasted unsalted almonds

- Chocolate chips, nuts, banana chips, dried fruit, vanilla, etc.

DIRECTIONS

1. Pulse dates before little pieces remain in the food processor. This should have the strength of the dough.

1. Optional second step: In a 350 Fahrenheit oven, toast the oats for 10 to 15 minutes or until golden brown. If you don't want to toast them, keep them raw.

2. In a wide mixing cup, combine the peas, almonds, and dates; set aside.

3. In a saucepan above low heat, melt the maple syrup & peanut butter. Stir & pour over the oat mixture, then stir to spread the dates equally.

4. Switch to an 8" baking dish or the other compact pan lined in parchment paper or plastic wrap so they can be quickly extracted.

5. Force down tightly until evenly flattened – then press down & stack the bars with something flat, similar to a drinking glass, which makes them stay together easier.

6. Cover with plastic wrap or parchment paper & ice or freeze for 15 to 20 minutes to firm up.

7. Detach bars from the pan and break into ten equal bars. For up to a few days, pack in the airtight jar.

NUTRITION: Calories: 231 kcal Fat: 9.7 g Protein: 5.8 g Carbs: 33.9 g

12. Eggplant Hash with eggs

Ready in: 20 minutes

Servings: 5

Difficulty: Easy

INGREDIENTS

- Black pepper to taste

- 2 tbsp olive oil

- 8 oz chopped cheese

- Salt to taste

- ½ chopped onion

- One sliced eggplant

- 4 tbsp butter

- Eight egg

- ½ tsp soy sauce

DIRECTIONS

The Execution

1. Add the olive oil & onion to the frying pan. Sauté till onion is soft.

2. Add the eggplant & halloumi cheese to the pan & cook till everything is golden brown, occasionally stirring—season with salt & pepper to taste. When finished, plate the hash & cover to keep warm.

3. Put the eggs over the eggplant hash. Serve with remaining butter from the pan & Worcestershire sauce. Season with additional salt & pepper if desired.

NUTRITION: Calories: 554 kcal Fat: 43.6 g Protein: 36.1 g Carbs: 6.0 g

13. Easy Nachos

Ready in: 25 minutes

Servings: 8

Difficulty: Easy

INGREDIENTS

- ½ cup Black olives

- One packet Tortilla Chips

- 1 cup Beef

- 1 lb cheese

- 1 cup Chopped chicken

- 1/3 cup Tomatoes chili

- ½ cup Beans

DIRECTIONS

1. Preheat oven to 350 Fahrenheit.

2. Line a baking sheet with foil.

3. Now spread chips over it.

4. Then you sprinkle 1/2 of the grated cheese over the chips.

5. Again sprinkle toppings over the chips & cheese.

6. Sprinkle now the remaining cheese.

7. Bake it for around 10 mins, or till cheese is melty good.

8. Serve it warm with sides such as sour cream or salsa.

NUTRITION: Calories: 447 kcal Fat: 26 g Protein: 17 g Carbs: 38 g

14. Homemade ketchup

Ready in: 12 hours 10 minutes

Servings: 48

Difficulty: Difficult

INGREDIENTS

- One clove

- 28 oz chopped tomatoes

- 2/3 cup sugar

- ½ cup water

- ¾ cup vinegar

- ½ tsp garlic paste

- 1 tsp onion paste

- Salt to taste

- Black pepper to taste

- 1/8 tsp mustard powder

DIRECTIONS

1. First of all, pour some ground tomatoes into a slow cooker. Swirl 1/4 cup of water in each emptied container & place it into the slow cooker. Add some sugar, celery salt, garlic powder, vinegar, onion powder, salt, black pepper, mustard powder, cayenne pepper, & whole clove; whisk to combine.

2. Cook it on high flame, uncovered, till mixture is reduced by 1/2 & very thick, 10- 12 hrs. Stir well every hr. or so.

3. Smooth this texture of ketchup using a blender, around 20 seconds.

4. Now shift the strained ketchup in a bowl. Cool it thoroughly before tasting to adjust salt, cayenne pepper/ black pepper.

NUTRITION: Calories: 16 kcal Fat: g Protein: 0.5 g Carbs: 3.9 g

15. Greek Tzatziki

Ready in: 15 minutes

Servings: 5

Difficulty: Easy

INGREDIENTS

- 1 tbsp dill

- ½ sliced cucumber

- 4 tbsp chopped garlic

- 1 ½ cup yogurt

- 2 tbsp olive oil

- Salt to taste

- 2 tbsp vinegar

DIRECTIONS

1. Firstly, grate the cucumber & drain it through a fine-mesh overnight in the fridge.

2. Now mix the yogurt, vinegar, garlic, oil, & salt in a wide bowl. Cover & refrigerate it overnight.

3. Now shifted this grated cucumber & fresh yogurt mixture & stir to combine. So now you serve it chilled with pita bread for dipping.

NUTRITION: Calories: 75 kcal Fat: 6 g Protein: 4 g Carbs: 3 g

Chapter 5: Soup Recipes

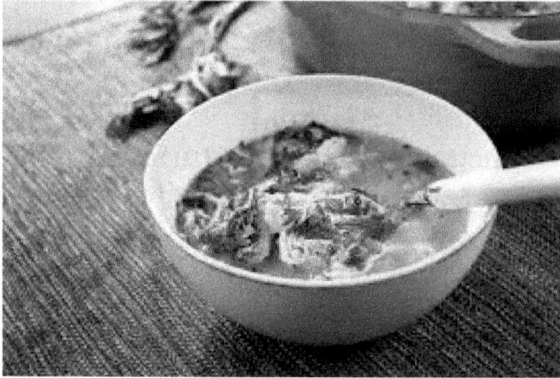

1. Beef Barley Vegetable Soup

Ready in: 360 minutes

Servings: 10

Difficulty: Easy

INGREDIENTS

- 3 lb beef

- One bay leaf

- ½ cup barley

- 2 tbsp oil

- Three diced celery stalk

- Three diced carrot

- One diced onion

- 4 cups water

- 16 oz mixed vegetables

- Black pepper as required

- Four cubes of bouillon

- 1 tbsp sugar

- 28 oz diced tomatoes

- ¼ tsp black pepper

- Salt as required

DIRECTIONS

1. For 5 hours, cook chuck roast in a slow cooker until it tender. Add bay and barley leaf in it when cooking reaches its last hour. Chop the meat into small pieces after removing it. Remove bay leaf and set the barley, beef, and broth aside.

2. On medium heat, heat oil in a wide stockpot. Cook carrots, onions, mixed vegetables, and celery until they tender. Add beef bouillon, water, sugar, pepper, chopped tomatoes, and barley mixture. Heat it until it boils, then reduce heat till it simmers for 20 minutes. To impart some more taste, use pepper and salt. Serve and enjoy the meal.

NUTRITION: Calories: 321 cal Fat: 17.3 g Protein: 20 g Carbs: 23 g

2. Hearty Vegetable Stew

Ready in: 60 minutes

Servings: 6

Difficulty: Medium

INGREDIENTS

Sauté Mixture

- Six minced garlic clove

- 3 tbsp olive oil

- Two sliced celery stalk

- One chopped onion

- Two diced carrots

Rouz mixture

- 4 cups vegetable stock

- Black pepper as required

- 1 tbsp chopped sage

- 1 tbsp chopped rosemary

- 1 tbsp chopped thyme

- ¼ cup wine

- ¼ cup rice flour

Vegetable stew

- 1 cup peas

- 2 cups chopped sweet potato

- 2 tbsp tomato paste

- Four chopped red potato

- 1 tsp marmite

- 1 tbsp soy sauce

- 1 tsp liquid smoke

- 1 tsp salt

- 1 tbsp yeast

- 2 tbsp wine

DIRECTIONS

1. Heat Olive oil in a pot over a medium flame and then add carrot, onion, and celery. Cook them until the onions are soft; it may take 9 minutes. Then add fresh herbs, garlic, and black pepper and cook again for almost 3 minutes.

2. Add flour and keep stirring to coat the added vegetables, cook for one more minute, and do not stop stirring. Now pour the white wine and add vegetable broth slowly with a quarter of a cup at a time. It is important to keep stirring to avoid lump formation between flour and liquid.

3. Stir the tomato paste, marmite, nutritional yeast, potato, liquid smoke, soy sauce, sweet potato, boil it gently, and then simmer. Cook, it uncovered for about 30 minutes until the vegetables are tendered and keep stirring while cooking.

4. Stir the red wine vinegar and frozen peas, and then set them to cook for about 6 minutes until the peas are tender. Sprinkle some salt and pepper to impart taste to the meal. Serve the product hot and enjoy the meal.

NUTRITION: Calories: 286 cal Fat: 7 g Protein: 7 g Carbs: 48 g

3. Butternut Squash Soup

Ready in: 50 minutes

Servings: 7

Difficulty: Easy

INGREDIENTS

- ½ cup coconut milk
- 2 cups vegetable broth
- One chopped carrot
- Four minced garlic clove
- One chopped smith apple
- One chopped onion
- ¼ tsp black pepper
- 3 lb chopped butternut squash
- One sage sprig
- ¼ tsp cinnamon
- ½ tsp salt
- 1/8 tsp cayenne pepper
- ¼ tsp nutmeg

DIRECTIONS

1. Add all the ingredients to the small slow cooker and heat them for 8 hours at low flame or heat until ingredients are tender and are capable of mashing with folk at ease. Abolish the sage and stir with coconut milk.

2. With the help of an immersion blender, puree soup to the point that it becomes smooth. Taste it and add salt or pepper as desired. Serve and enjoy the meal.

NUTRITION: Calories: 305 cal Fat: 6.8 g Protein: 6.9 g Carbs: 60 g

4. Chicken Cordon Blew Soup

Ready in: 20 minutes

Servings: 8

Difficulty: Easy

INGREDIENTS

- 3 cups chicken stock

- ¼ cup butter

- One minced garlic clove

- ½ chopped onion

- ¼ cup flour

- 2 cups half and half

- 8 oz cream cheese

- 2 cup chicken, rotisserie

- One ¼ cup grated cheese, Swiss

- 1 cup chopped ham

DIRECTIONS

1. Take a large pot, melt butter in it, and then add diced onion in it. Cook until the onion gets soften. Then add garlic and heat the mixture for 1 minute, followed by flour, and put it for one more minute.

2. Draw chicken pieces into the pot slowly and add cream cheese into the pot and stir it. Stir Swiss cheese until it gets melted. Stir the ham and chicken until heated. Now serve the meal hot and enjoy it.

NUTRITION: Calories: 507 cal Fat: 26 g Protein: 34 g Carbs: 37 g

5. Swedish Meatballs with Cream of Mushroom Soup

Ready in: 35 minutes

Servings: 6

Difficulty: Easy

INGREDIENTS

Meatballs

- One egg

- ½ cup bread crumbs

- 2 tbsp olive oil

- One diced onion

- 1 tbsp diced parsley

- ½ lb lean pork

- 1 lb lean beef

- ¼ cup milk

- 1 tsp salt

- ¼ tsp nutmeg

- ½ tsp garlic powder

- 1/8 tsp allspice

- ¼ tsp black pepper

For frying

- 1 tbsp Worcestershire sauce

- 1 tbsp olive oil

- Mushroom Sauce

- 2 tbsp butter

- 1 cup beef stock

- ¼ cup sour cream

- 1 cup mushroom cream soup

DIRECTIONS

1. Take a large-sized skillet, and on medium heat, roast crumbs of bread while stirring it continuously. The toasty smell and dark brown color of bread will indicate that it has been roasted. Now transfer it to a large mixing bowl.

2. Now heat Olive oil in the skillet and add and cook onions in it for three minutes. Sprinkle a salt pinch and pepper to impart taste and move it to the bowl of breadcrumbs.

3. Now add milk, parsley, ground meat, egg, spices, and salt to the onion and bread crumb mixture. Mesh the mixture well.

4. Convert the meat mixture in the form of meatballs of some even size. Place them on a plate and set them aside.

5. On medium heat, melt butter and oil in a skillet. Now cook the meatballs in till they turn brown.

6. Now to clean the skillet, pour the broth and bring it to a boil so that stirring could help remove these scraps from the bottom of the skillet. If you are using a non-stick pan, it won't be an issue then.

7. Now stir the sour and mushroom cream.

8. Then put back the meatball into the pan and mitigate the heat and cook it for 6 minutes.

9. Your meatballs are ready now and serve them while they are hot. Serve them with noodles, and never forget to pour sauce and sprinkle parsley over it. Serve and enjoy the meal.

NUTRITION: Calories: 409 kcal Fat: 10 g Protein: 27 g Carbs: 12 g

6. Swedish Meatballs Soup

Ready in: 50 minutes

Servings: 6

Difficulty: Easy

INGREDIENTS

Meatballs

- ¼ cup diced parsley

- 1 lb beef

- ½ cup ricotta cheese

- 1 lb ground turkey

- Two eggs

- 1 tsp salt

- ½ cup breadcrumbs

- ½ tsp pepper

- ¼ tsp nutmeg

- ¼ tsp allspice

Soup

- 8 oz pasta

- One sliced onion

- 1/3 cup flour

- 6 tbsp butter

- ½ tsp nutmeg

- 6 cups beef broth

- ½ tsp allspice

- ½ cup heavy cream

- Salt to taste

- 1 cup sour cream

- Black pepper to taste

- 2 tbsp diced parsley

- Dill weed as required

DIRECTIONS

1. Heat oven up to 400 Fahrenheit.

2. Now mix the ingredients of the meatball in a bowl.

3. Form the mixture into the size of walnut balls and put the meatballs into the baking dish. Bake them for 25 minutes until they are cooked.

4. Cook onion in melted butter in a Dutch Oven of large size until they are tender. Then remove them from the pot.

5. Stir Spices, flour, and the nutmeg in the butter remained behind and cooked for 2 minutes.

6. Pour broth and cook it while stirring until it gets thickened. Add meatballs and bring them to a simmer.

7. Now follow the instructions on package cook pasta.

8. Along with heavy sour cream and parsley, stir the pasta into the pot. Season the meat with pepper and salt according to your taste.

9. Fill the bowl with soup and serve it hot and enjoy it.

NUTRITION: Calories: 656 cal Fat: 31.5 g Protein: 30 g Carbs: 60.5 g

7. Potato Cauliflower and Ham Soup

Ready in: 35 minutes

Servings: 5

Difficulty: Easy

INGREDIENTS

- 1 cup grated cheese

- 5 ½ cups diced cauliflower

- 2 cups diced broccoli

- 5 cups chopped russet potatoes

- 1 tsp salt

- 1/3 cup chopped celery

- 8 cups water

- 5 cups chopped ham, cooked

- 6 tbsp flour

- 4 tbsp chicken bouillon

- 6 tbsp butter

- 2 ½ cups milk

- 2 tsp black pepper

DIRECTIONS

1. Mix all the ingredients in a stockpot. Boil the ingredients and then cover the pot and mitigate the heat level. Boil them for 12 minutes until they are soft. Stir it in the pepper, chicken bouillon, and salt. With the help of a fork, break cauliflower and potatoes into small pieces.

2. Melt the butter in a separate saucepan at medium heat. Add Sweep flour in it and cook for 2 minutes until the mixture gets thick. Now stir it in the cheese and milk for 6 minutes.

3. Stir the mixture of milk in the stockpot and then cook the soup.

4. Then garnish it with cheddar cheese.

NUTRITION: Calories: 257 cal Fat: 10 g Protein: 21 g Carbs: 6 g

8. Chicken Tortilla Soup

Ready in: 40 minutes

Servings: 8

Difficulty: Easy

INGREDIENTS

- 1 cup corn

- 1 tbsp olive oil

- Three minced garlic clove

- One diced onion

- One chopped jalapeno

- 1 tsp chili powder

- 1 tsp cumin

- 14 ½ oz mashed tomatoes

- 3 cup chicken stock

- 2 tbsp lime juice

- 2 cups chopped tomatoes

- 14 ½ oz black beans

- 2 lb chicken boneless pieces

- ¼ cup diced cilantro

- One diced avocado

DIRECTIONS

1. Heat Olive oil at medium heat in a pan. Add and fry tortilla strips in stages until they are crisp, and then drain it and sprinkle with a salt pinch.

2. Now at medium flame, heat olive oil, add jalapeno, onion, and garlic, and cook them until they get soft.

3. Add all the ingredients which remained behind and let it simmer for 25 minutes, or the chicken is cooked.

4. Remove and shred the chicken, and then add it back into the stockpot and let it simmer for 4 minutes.

5. Pour the soup into the bowl and mix it with sliced avocado, tortilla strips, and lime wedges.

NUTRITION: Calories: 278 cal Fat: 11 g Protein: 18 g Carbs: 27 g

9. Mulligatawny Soup

Ready in: 80 minutes

Servings: 6

Difficulty: Medium

INGREDIENTS

- ½ cup heavy cream

- ½ cup diced onion

- One chopped carrot

- Two diced celery stalks

- ¼ cup butter

- 1 ½ tsp curry powder

- 1 ½ tbsp all-purpose flour

- 4 cups chicken stock

- ¼ cup rice

- ½ chopped apple

- 2 lb chicken boneless pieces

- Salt to taste

- ¼ tsp thyme, dried

- Black pepper to taste

DIRECTIONS

1. Cook onions, carrot, butter, and celery in the pot of soup. Then add curry and flour and then cook it for 6 minutes. Further, add in chicken stock and boil and let it simmer for half an hour.

2. Now add rice, salt, thyme, rice, and salt, and then let it get cooked for 20 minutes.

3. Add hot cream and then serve it hot and enjoy.

NUTRITION: Calories: 223 cal Fat: 15.8 g Protein: 7 g Carbs: 13.5 g

10. Egg and Lemon Soup

Ready in: 90 minutes

Servings: 6

Difficulty: Difficult

INGREDIENTS

- ¼ cup Lemon juice

- 1 kg Chicken

- One chopped onion

- Black pepper to taste

- 8 cup water

- ½ cup chopped orzo

- Salt to taste

- Four egg

For Serving

- Black pepper

- Oregano

- ½ lemon

DIRECTIONS

1. Bake chicken, and it is stock with peppercorns chicken, salt, water, and onion, and baked chicken for 60 minutes. Then strain the chicken broth, and shred them into pieces to the chicken. Now bake orzo in the broth for 9 to 20 minutes; after that, made the avgolemono by placing the egg in lemon juice and add into the soup. Then mix the avgolemono into chicken orzo and stir to combine it, thicken it for 3 to minutes, and don't boil. Serve it with a lemon slice, oregano, and black pepper.

NUTRITION: Calories: 431 kcal Fat: 28.2 g Protein: 30.7 g Carbs: 12.8 g

11. Seafood Bisque

Ready in: 30 minutes

Servings: 10

Difficulty: Easy

INGREDIENTS

- Onion to chopped

- Two can Mushroom soup

- 3 tbsp chicken soup

- Two cups of celery soup

- 6 oz crabmeat

- 2 2/3 cup milk

- Four crushed onion

- 11/2 lb chopped shrimp

- ½ crushed celery

Pepper to taste

- One clove chopped Garlic

- ¼ tsp chili sauce

- 1 tsp sauce

DIRECTIONS

1. mix all eight components, boil them, combine shrimp, mushrooms, and carbs and boil it for 9 to 20 minutes. Mix them in wine, salt, and pepper and cook for 2 to 3 minutes. Serve online and enjoy.

NUTRITION: Calories: 169 kcal Fat: 6 g Protein: 18 g Carbs: 10 g

12. Sausage Potato and Kale Soup

Ready in: 60 minutes

Servings: 12

Difficulty: Medium

INGREDIENTS

- 1 lb Italian sausage

- 2 cups kale leaves

- 4 cups cream (half and a half)

- ½ tsp black pepper

- ½ tsp red Chili

- 3 cups chopped tomatoes

- ½ tsp chopped Oregano

- 2 cups chicken soup

- One crushed onion

- 2 cups milk

DIRECTIONS

1. In a pot, add crumble sausage and cook it for 8 minutes. Combine red pepper flakes, potatoes, oregano, chicken broth, onion, and milk and boil them for half an hour. Serve with black pepper after boiling for 15 minutes.

NUTRITION: Calories: 266 kcal Fat: 18 g Protein: 10.6 g Carbs: 16.4 g

13. Seafood Cioppino

Ready in: 165 minutes

Servings: 8

Difficulty: Difficult

INGREDIENTS

- 1 lb Cod Fillets

- ¼ cup olive oil

- 10 oz scallops

- One crushed onion

- 25 shrimp

- Four cloves chopped garlic

- 25 mussels, drained

- One crushed bell pepper

- 10 oz clam juice

- 1 cup wine

- One green chili

- ½ crushed Parsley

- 1 tsp cayenne Pepper

- Salt to taste

- 1 tsp Paprika

- Black pepper to taste

- 2 tsp chopped basil

- ½ cup water

- 1 tsp chopped oregano

- 1 tsp thyme

- One can of tomato sauce

- Two cups of chopped tomatoes

DIRECTIONS

1. In a pan cook oil, with pepper, onion, bell pepper, and garlic; mix the juice of calm, parsley, cayenne pepper, salt, paprika, pepper, water, basil, tomato sauce, oregano, thyme, and tomatoes, and boil for 60 to 120 minutes. Finally, combine scallops, clams, cod, prawns, and mussels and mix serve and enjoy it.

NUTRITION: Calories: 303 kcal Fat: 9.1 g Protein: 34.3 g Carbs: 16.5 g

14. Turkey chili Taco Soup

Ready in: 20 minutes

Servings: 9

Difficulty: Easy

INGREDIENTS

- 2 ½ chicken soup

- 1.3 lb grounded Turkey

- One packet taco seasoning

- 16 oz beans

- One crushed Onion

- One crushed bell pepper

- 8 oz tomato sauce

- 10 oz tomatoes chili

- 15 oz Kidney Beans

- 15 oz chopped frozen corn

DIRECTIONS

1. in a pan, cook onion in oil for 4 minutes, mix taco seasoning tomatoes, bean, corn, and chicken broth, and boil them for 16 to 20 minutes. Serve the soup with topping like fat sour cream, cheese, onions.

NUTRITION: Calories: 225 kcal Fat: 2 g Protein: 22 g Carbs: 31.5 g

Chapter 6: Salad Recipes

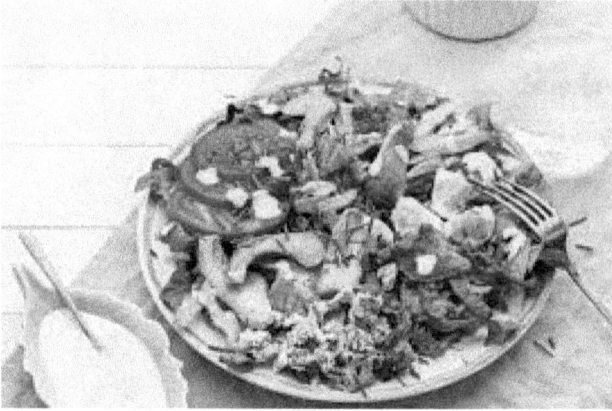

1. Green beans and Heart of Palm

Ready in 20 minutes

Servings: 8

Difficulty: Easy

INGREDIENTS

- ½ cup of chopped basil

- 1 lb. green beans

- 1 cup olives

- 1-1/2 cups of sliced palms

- ¾ crumbled cheese

- One lemon juice

- ½ cup of chopped oregano

- 1tbsp vinegar

- 1/3 cup of olive oil

DIRECTIONS

1. Boil green beans in salted water for 3-4 minutes. Drain and keep aside to cool.

2. Mix the vinegar, olive oil, oregano, basil, and lemon juice to make the dressing.

3. Take a large bowl and mix all the ingredients.

4. Toss well.

5. Serve and enjoy.

NUTRITION: Calories: 40 cal Fat: 3 g Protein: 4 g Carbs: 5 g

2. Crab Pasta

Ready in: 10 minutes

Servings: 4

Difficulty: Easy

INGREDIENTS

- 3 tbsp of olive oil

- 225g pasta

- Handful of parsley

- Red pepper flakes

- 225g crabmeat

- One garlic clove

DIRECTIONS

1. Boil pasta according to the given instructions. Drain and keep aside.

2. Chop parsley leaves.

3. Cook garlic in 2-3 tbsp olive oil in a saucepan.

4. At low heat, add pasta, crab meat, and all other ingredients and cook till all the ingredients are well mixed and softened.

5. Season with red pepper flakes.

6. Serve and enjoy.

NUTRITION: Calories: 311 cal Fat: 21 g Protein: 22 g Carbs: 6 g

3. Eggplant Salad

Ready in: 25 minutes

Servings: 2

Difficulty: Easy

INGREDIENTS

- Two garlic cloves

- Two sized eggplant

- 1-1/2 tsp salt and pepper

- One diced tomato

- 1-1/2 tsp red wine vinegar

- 3 tbsp olive oil

- ½ tsp chopped oregano

- Pita bread to serve

- Capers

DIRECTIONS

1. Take a grill and heat over medium flame. Place eggplant and prick with a fork and cook for 10-15 minutes till the skin is blistered.

2. Scoop out the eggplant.

3. Take a large bowl and mix all the ingredients.

4. Season with salt and pepper.

5. Use capers to garnish.

6. Serve with bread.

7. Enjoy.

NUTRITION: Calories: 156 cal Fat: 95 g Protein: 1.8 g Carbs: 16 g

4. Creamy Cucumber Salad

Ready in: 10 minutes

Servings: 8

Difficulty: Easy

INGREDIENTS

- ½ tsp of sugar

- 2-3 cucumbers

- ½ cup of sour cream

- 1/3 sliced onions

- ¼ cup chopped dill

- Salt to taste

- 3 tbsp white vinegar

DIRECTIONS

1. Peel and cut the cucumbers.

2. Take a large bowl and combine all the ingredients.

3. Toss well and refrigerate for 50-60 minutes.

4. Serve and enjoy.

NUTRITION: Calories: 77 cal Fat: 7 g Protein: 1 g Carbs: 4 g

5. Spinach with Egg and Bacon

Ready in: 10 minutes

Servings: 6

Difficulty: Easy

INGREDIENTS

- Six eggs

- 480 g cherry tomatoes

- 1tbsp olive oil

- 250g bacon

- 240g spinach

- Six toasted bread slices

- 1tbsp white vinegar

DIRECTIONS

1. Take a baking dish.

2. Put baking paper sprayed with oil and palace tomatoes in it.

3. Bake them in preheated oven for 20-25 minutes.

4. Take a pan and cook bacon for 2-3 minutes.

5. Transfer it to the plate.

6. Now cook spinach with 1 tbsp of olive oil in the pan for 2-3 minutes.

7. Boil water, adds a spoon of vinegar and carefully crack the egg in a separate small bowl and drop in the pan's middle.

8. Cook all the eggs and transfer them to the six serving plates.

9. Top with remaining ingredients.

10. Season with salt and black pepper.

11. Serve and enjoy.

NUTRITION: Calories: 55 Cal Fat: 15 g Protein: 21 g Carbs: 4 g

6. Buffalo Chicken Salad

Ready in: 60 minutes

Servings: 4

Difficulty: moderate

INGREDIENTS

Meat ingredients

- 2tbsp honey

- 1cup buffalo sauce

- Salt

- 1tbsp olive oil

- 1 lb. boneless chicken

- Black pepper

- ½ tsp onion powder

- One lime juice

- 1 tsp garlic powder

Dressing ingredients

- ½ tsp. black pepper

- ½ cup mayonnaise

- 1/2 cup buttermilk

- ½ cream

- ¼ cup chopped parsley

- Two minced garlic cloves

- ½ tbsp salt

- 2 tbsp chopped chives

- Cayenne pepper

Salad ingredients

- ¼ cup crumbled cheese

- 4 cup chopped romaine

- Two sliced celery

- 2 cup spinach

- One carrot

- ½ sliced onion

- One cucumber

- 1 cup cherry tomatoes

DIRECTIONS

1. Take a large bowl and mix meat, honey, lemon juice, onion, and garlic powder. Add salt and pepper to taste.

2. Add chicken meat to marinade.

3. Toss well.

4. Keep aside for 25-30 minutes at room temperature.

5. Heat oil in a skillet over medium flame and cook chicken for 10-20 minutes.

6. Place the cooked chicken on a chopping board and make small pieces of it.

7. Take a bowl and mix mayonnaise, cream & buttermilk. Put other ingredients and stir well.

8. Keep in the refrigerator for 50 minutes.

9. Mix all the salad ingredients in a large bowl.

10. Top the salad with cooked chicken and serve.

11. Enjoy.

NUTRITION: Calories: 291 cal Fat: 10.8 g Protein: 31.6g Carbs: 15 g

7. Cobb Egg Salad

Ready in: 20 minutes

Servings: 6

Difficulty: Easy

INGREDIENTS

- Eight crumbled bacon strips

- 3 tbsp. mayonnaise

- 3tbsp. yogurt

- Salt to taste

- 2-3 tbsp red wine vinegar

- Eight boiled eggs

- pepper to taste

- One sliced avocado

- ½ cherry tomatoes

- ½ crumbled cheese

- 2 tbsp chopped chives

DIRECTIONS

1. Take a bowl and mix mayonnaise, vinegar, and yogurt.

2. Sprinkle salt and pepper.

3. Mix the remaining ingredients in a large bowl.

4. Add mayonnaise mixture.

5. Mix well.

6. Garnish with chopped chives.

7. Serve and enjoy.

NUTRITION: Calories: 235 cal Fat: 16.7 g Protein: 13.5 g Carbs: 8.8 g

8. Chinese Chicken Salad

Ready in: 15 minutes

Servings: 3

Difficulty: Easy

INGREDIENTS

Dressing ingredients

- 2 tbsp soy sauce

- 1tbsp toasted sesame oil

- 3 tbsp of rice vinegar

- One garlic clove

- 2 tbsp of grapeseed oil

- 1-1/2 tsp minced ginger

- 1 tsp of sugar

- ½ tsp of pepper

Salad ingredients

- 1 cup of carrot

- 4 cups of cabbage

- Two cups of chicken

- 1-1/2 cups of red cabbage

- ½ cups of shallots

Garnishes

- 2-3 tsp of sesame seeds

- ½ cup of crunchy noodles

DIRECTIONS

1. Take a jar and gently mix the dressing ingredients and keep aside for 10-15 minutes.

2. Take a large bowl and mix the salad ingredients with crunchy noodles.

3. Drizzle with dressing.

4. Toss well.

5. Distribute in the serving bowls and garnish with crunchier noodles.

6. Serve and enjoy.

NUTRITION: Calories: 412 cal Fat: 23.2 g Protein: 32.3 g Carbs: 17.3 g

9. Loaded Italian Salad

Ready in: 20 minutes

Servings: 3

Difficulty: Easy

INGREDIENTS

- ¼ cup of water

- One pack Italian mix dressing

- Half tsp sugar

- ½ tsp Italian dried seasoning

- 1/3 tsp garlic powder

- 1/3 cup of white vinegar

- ¾ cup of vegetable oil

- ½ tsp salt

- pepper

- ½ tbsp of mayonnaise

DIRECTIONS

1. Take a bowl and mix all the ingredients.

2. Shake well to combine.

3. Serve and enjoy.

NUTRITION: Calories: 630 cal Fat: 35 g Protein: 29 g Carbs: 49 g

10. Dill Cucumber Salad

Ready in: 1:00-15 minutes

Servings: 8

Difficulty: Easy

INGREDIENTS

- 2 tsp red wine vinegar

- One lb cucumbers

- 2 tsp salt

- ½ peeled red onions

- 2 tsp sugar

- 2 tsp balsamic vinegar

- ½ cup of water

- 2 tsp apple cider vinegar

- ¼ cup of chopped dill leaves

DIRECTIONS

1. Take a bowl and mix sliced cucumbers, salt, sugar, and pepper. Place in the fridge for 60 minutes.

2. Take out from the refrigerator and drain.

3. Add other ingredients and mix.

4. Serve and enjoy.

NUTRITION: Calories: 16 cal Fat: 1 g Protein: 1 g Carbs: 3 g

11. Cucumber Avocado Salad with Lime Mint and Feta

Ready in: 35 minutes

Servings: 4

Difficulty: Easy

INGREDIENTS

- 2-3 chopped avocados

- 2 cups of chopped cucumbers

- ½ cup of chopped mint

- Pinch of salt

- One lime juice

- ½ cup of crumbled feta

For dressing

- 1 tbsp lime juice

- 2 tbsp olive oil

DIRECTIONS

1. Cut the cucumbers.

2. Season with salt and pepper. Keep aside for 30-35 minutes.

3. Drain them and add olive oil and lime juice.

4. Mix well.

5. Mix all the ingredients in a large bowl.

6. Add dressing and mix well.

7. Serve and enjoy.

NUTRITION: Calories: 289 cal Fat: 26 g Protein: 5 g Carbs: 14 g

12. Avocado Egg Salad

Ready in: 25 minutes

Servings: 2

Difficulty: Easy

INGREDIENTS

- Lettuce leaves

- One diced avocado

- 2tbsp chopped red onion

- Three boiled eggs

- 1 tbsp chopped chives

- 2tbsp mayonnaise

- Salt

- 1 tbsp chopped parsley

- 1tsp lemon juice

- pepper to taste

DIRECTIONS

1. Take a large bowl and mix all the ingredients.

2. Serve with bread topped with lettuce leaves.

3. Enjoy.

NUTRITION: Calories: 119 cal Fat: 8.7 g Protein: 7.2 g Carbs: 3.4 g

13. Red Cabbage and Egg Salad

Ready in: 30 minutes

Servings: 3

Difficulty: Easy

INGREDIENTS

- ½ tsp salt

- Five diced carrots

- ½ red cabbage

- Four boiled eggs

- One red pepper-small

- ½ chopped parsley

- One chopped red onion

- pepper

For dressing

- 1 tsp ground sugar

- 2 tbsp of mayonnaise

- 3-4 tbsp yogurt

- 1 tbsp apple cider vinegar

- 1-2 tbsp salad cream

DIRECTIONS

1. Cut the cabbage.

2. Take a large mixing bowl and mix diced boiled eggs, cabbage, dressing, and other remaining ingredients.

3. Add parsley.

4. Mix well.

5. Serve and enjoy.

NUTRITION: Calories: 199 cal Fat: 8.9 g Protein: 14.6 g Carbs: 19.9 g

14. Strawberry Jello

Ready in: 40 minutes

Servings: 10

Difficulty: Easy

INGREDIENTS

- Nine oz. mix strawberry jello

- Eight oz. cooled whip

- One lb. strawberries

DIRECTIONS

1. Take mix jello powder and one cup of boiling water in a large mixing bowl followed by 1-cup cold water.

2. Stir well till the jello is melted.

3. Place it in the refrigerator.

4. Let the mixture set well.

5. Add cooled whip and stir so that everything combines well.

6. Take a springform pan and spray it with oil. Add the mixture in it and place halved strawberries on the top.

7. Refrigerate for 30 minutes.

8. Mix 1-cup of boiled water and 3oz. Strawberry jello in a separate jar.

9. Refrigerate.

10. Put the jello mixture on the top and allow it to set.

11. Serve and enjoy.

NUTRITION: Calories: 121 cal Fat: 1 g Protein: 2 g Carbs: 27 g

15. Mac Cheeseburger Salad

Ready in: 20 minutes. minutes

Servings: 4

Difficulty: Easy

INGREDIENTS

- 1 cup cheddar

- 1 lb ground beef

- 1 tbsp of Worcestershire sauce

- Salt and ground pepper

- 1 tbsp red wine vinegar

- 1 tsp of garlic powder

- ½ cup yogurt

- One sliced tomato

- 1 tsp ketchup

- 2 tsp mustard

- ½ tsp paprika

- Two chopped lettuce

- 1 tsp sesame seeds

- ¼ sliced onion

- Quartered dill pickle

DIRECTIONS

1. Take a skillet and heat over medium flame. Add beef, sauce, salt, garlic powder, and pepper. Cook for 5-10 minutes.

2. For the dressing, mix yogurt, mustard, vinegar, paprika, and ketchup in a large bowl.

3. Assembly: mix tomatoes, romaine, pickles, onions, and cheddar in a large mixing bowl. Add dressing.

4. Use sesame seeds for garnishing.

5. Serve and enjoy.

NUTRITION: Calories: 368 cal Fat: 31 g Protein: 18 g Carbs: 3 g

Chapter 7: Smoothies Recipes

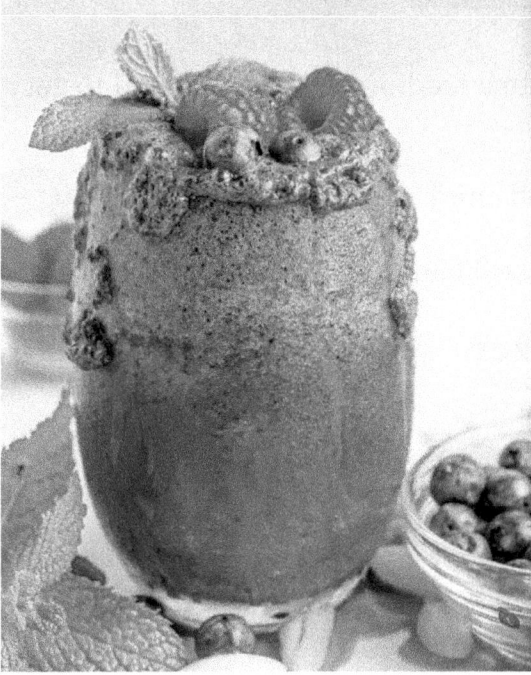

1. Frappe

Ready in: 5 minutes

Servings: 1

Difficulty: Easy

INGREDIENTS

- Ice cubes as required

- 1 ½ cup chilled coffee

- 2 tbsp sugar syrup

- ½ cup milk

- Whipped cream for serving as required

DIRECTIONS

1. Add all the ingredients to a food processor and blend to get a smooth, creamy mixture.

2. Serve with ice cream and enjoy it.

NUTRITION: Calories: 89 kcal Fat: 2 g Protein: 2 g Carbs: 16 g

2. White Wine Spritzer

Ready in: 5 minutes

Servings: 1

Difficulty: Easy

INGREDIENTS

- Lime slices for garnishing

- ¼ cup soda, chilled

- ¾ cup white wine, chilled

DIRECTIONS

1. Add wine and soda to a wine glass and stir well.

2. Serve and enjoy it.

NUTRITION: Calories: 90 cal Fat: 0 g Protein: 0 g Carbs: 3 g

3. Paloma

Ready in: 5 minutes

Servings: 1

Difficulty: Easy

INGREDIENTS

- ¼ oz sugar syrup

- 2 oz tequila

- 2 oz water, sparkling

- 2 oz grapefruit juice

- 4 tbsp lime juice

- Ice cubes as required

- Salt to taste

DIRECTIONS

1. Add all the ingredients to a food processor and blend to get a smooth mixture.

2. Serve and enjoy it.

NUTRITION: Calories: 212 cal Fat: 0 g Protein: 0 g Carbs: 17 g

4. Cherry Lime Slush

Ready in: 5 minutes

Servings: 2

Difficulty: Easy

INGREDIENTS

- ½ cup sugar

- 4 cups cherries, sweet

- 2 cups sparkling water

- ½ cup lime juice

DIRECTIONS

1. Add all the ingredients to a food processor and blend to get a smooth mixture.

2. Serve and enjoy it.

NUTRITION: Calories: 189 kcal Fat: 1 g Protein: 3 g Carbs: 49 g

5. Caipirinha Cocktail

Ready in: 5 minutes

Servings: 1

Difficulty: Easy

INGREDIENTS

- 1 tbsp lime juice

- 1 ½ sliced lime

- 2 oz cachaça

- 2 tbsp sugar

- Crushed ice

DIRECTIONS

1. Add all the ingredients to a food processor and blend to get a smooth mixture.

2. Serve and enjoy it.

NUTRITION: Calories: 196 kcal Fat: 0.5 g Protein: 0.7 g Carbs: 11.2 g

6. Ginger Peach Vodka Mule

Ready in: 5 minutes

Servings: 2

Difficulty: Easy

INGREDIENTS

- 1 cup seltzer water

- 1 tsp ginger paste

- 2 oz peach syrup

- 2 oz vodka

DIRECTIONS

1. Add all the ingredients to a food processor and blend to get a smooth mixture.

2. Serve and enjoy it.

NUTRITION: Calories: 216 cal Fat: 1 g Protein: 0 g Carbs: 31 g

7. Starbucks Pink Drink

Ready in: 5 minutes

Servings: 4

Difficulty: Easy

INGREDIENTS

- Strawberry slices

- 1 cup tea, herbal

- ½ cup grape juice

- 1 cup boiling water

- 1 ½ cup coconut milk

DIRECTIONS

1. Add tea bags in cups and pour in boiling water. Remove the tea bags.

2. Add grape juice, ice, and coconut milk.

3. Place strawberry slices and serve.

NUTRITION: Calories: 124 cal Fat: 5 g Protein: 2 g Carbs: 21 g

8. Honeysuckle Iced Tea

Ready in: 15 minutes

Servings: 2

Difficulty: Easy

INGREDIENTS

- Honey as required

- Two ¼ cups honeysuckle flower

- 2 cups water

- Mint as required for garnishing

DIRECTIONS

1. Boil water in the pan and turn off the flame.

2. Add flowers in boiling water and stir.

3. Cover the pan and leave it for two hours.

4. Strain the flower-soaked water and discard the debris.

5. The honeysuckle is ready.

6. You can store it in an airtight container in the fridge.

7. Add honeysuckle in glass and add in ice.

8. Stir and serve.

NUTRITION: Calories: 69 cal Fat: 0 g Protein: 0 g Carbs: 9 g

9. Chocolate Caramel Delight Smoothie

Ready in: 10 minutes

Servings: 1

Difficulty: Easy

INGREDIENTS

- 2 tbsp grated toasted coconut

- 1 cup almond milk

- 1/3 cup chocolate shake

- 1 cup crushed ice

- 1 tsp caramel extract

DIRECTIONS

1. Add all the ingredients to a food processor and blend to get a smooth mixture.

2. Serve and enjoy it.

NUTRITION: Calories: 281 cal Fat: 12 g Protein: 19 g Carbs: 22 g

Conclusion

Everyone wants to have a safe, disease-free body. Physical activity, a healthy lifestyle, and a well-balanced diet are the most important ways to maintain optimal health. A ketogenic diet is the most common lifestyle trend today. This diet may seem to be at odds because the Keto diet reduces carbs to 20 to 25 g per day. The Keto diet is a low-carbohydrate, high-fat, moderate-protein diet that excludes many dairy products. Ingredients for a vegetable-based Ketogenic diet include low-carb vegetables, almonds and seeds and nuts, vegan protein sources, coconut, beans, and essential oils.

When following a Ketogenic diet, high-carb foods, including sweetened beverages, starchy vegetables (including potatoes, peas, and turnips), and grains, should be avoided. To ensure that dietary requirements are met, certain minerals and vitamins, such as iron, vitamin B12, and vitamin D, should be consumed.

Overall a ketogenic diet provides advantages in weight loss and reductions in overall cholesterol, blood pressure, and blood sugar in individuals. However, as opposed to the outcomes of traditional weight-loss diets, these effects after a year might not be substantially different. Some people that have struggled to lose weight with other strategies can benefit from a ketogenic diet. Because of the genetic makeup and body structure which differ from person to person, the exact ratio of fat, carb, and protein necessary to obtain health benefits also differs. Suppose someone decides to begin a ketogenic diet. In that case, it is advised to consult with a dietitian or physician to closely observe any metabolic modifications that occur after beginning the diet and develop a meal schedule that is personalized to one's current health needs to avoid nutritional shortages or other health problems. When you have lost weight, a dietitian can advise you about reintroducing carbohydrates in later diet stages.

CPSIA information can be obtained
at www.ICGtesting.com
Printed in the USA
BVHW050023090421
604476BV00005B/1259

9 781802 261783